Alessandra Moro Buronzo & Isabelle Brette

D1440267

Food healing
fruits – vegetables – spices

Their daily virtues

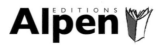

EDITIONS
Alpen

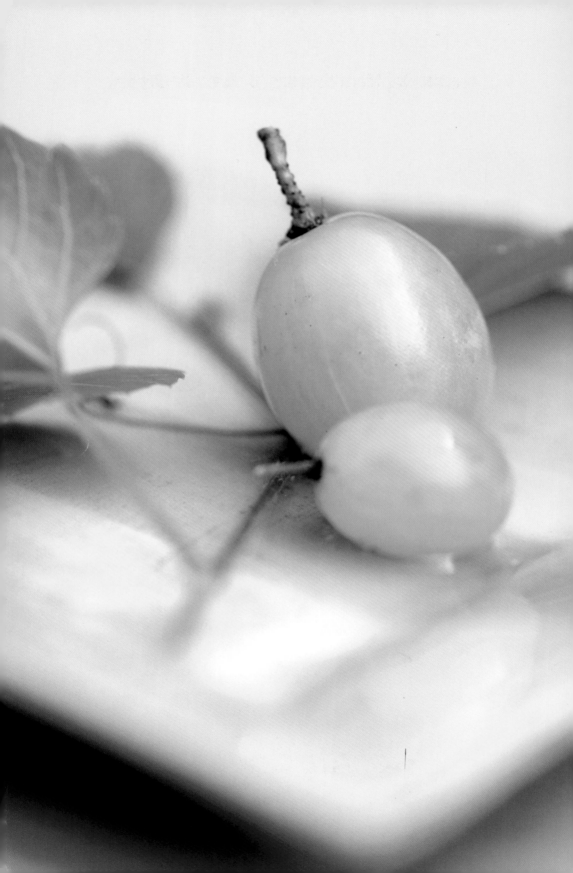

Alessandra Moro Buronzo & Isabelle Brette

Food healing
fruits - vegetables - spices

Their daily virtues

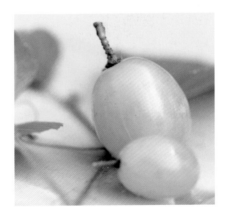

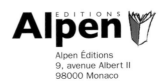

EDITIONS
Alpen

Alpen Éditions
9, avenue Albert II
98000 Monaco

Elizabeth Brette is a biochemist who has worked at the Nice hospital in France for 15 years. She is now the principal editor of the weekly "Journal Méditerranéen de la Santé".

A naturopath, Alessandra Moro Buronzo lives in Paris where she has worked for the past 18 years. She has had a keen interest in well-being issues and natural methods of healing for many years now. This passion and her interest in writing have brought her to laying on paper both her great knowledge and her many tips for a healthy living. She is a general press writer as well.

For the present edition
© 2011, Alpen Éditions
9, avenue Albert II
MC - 98000 MONACO
Tél. : 00377 97 77 62 10
Fax : 00377 97 77 62 11

Chief Editor: Christophe Didierlaurent
Editorial Board: Fabienne Desmarets
Desktop Publishing:
Stéphane Falaschi

Photo Credits:
Banana Stock, Corbis, Image State, Inspirestock, Photo Alto, Zen Shui

Copyright: 2011
ISBN13 : 978-235934-076-1

Printed in Italy
Papergraf press

INTRODUCTION

A healthy balanced diet is certainly a key to enabling us to stay fit and enjoy good health all through life.
If we had kept closer to our instinct, like animals have, we would know perfectly well what we need to eat.
Unfortunately, we have gradually lost this instinct and have ended up being overwhelmed by the number of products created and offered by the food industry thereby creating in us many false needs.
Indeed, in our industrialized countries, we have a very large number of foods at our disposal in often very large amounts.
But some are available out of their original seasons, others have been industrially modified.
Thus, we often eat foods that are too salty, too fatty, too sweet, too complicated, too polluted ...
Shying away from the famous phrase of Hippocrates, the father of modern medicine: «Let food be your only remedy! », food may now become a poison for our body.

Thankfully, it would seem that Americans care more and about the quality of what's on their plate. They seem to have understood that we must return to food that is more «natural» and less artificial.
Indeed, if inadequate or excessive intake of some nutrients may be the cause of certain diseases, intake of «good» foods may be the smartest strategy in the fight against many health problems.
Our habits must change, even if not by much...

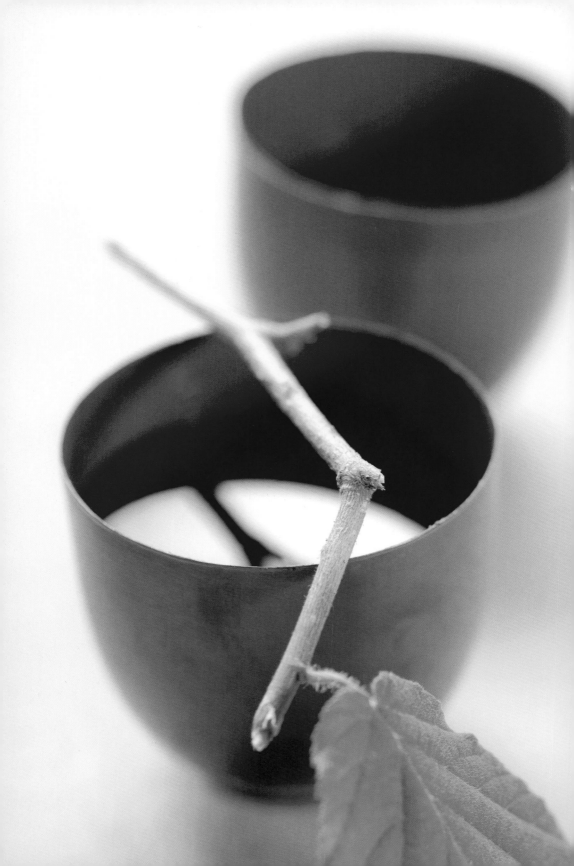

It is necessary to be detached when bombarded by commercials, thereby removing bad habits and getting closer to foods that help us get healthily nourished.
Let's take a step back when looking at industrial marketing let's bring common sense back into our lives!
And faced with the difficulties we may feel when we're trying to sort out the wealth of information often contradictory that is given to us daily, let's not throw in the towel.
Healthy foods are available to us and really, we do not need too much food to maintain a good capital (of) health; we just need to know what to eat.
In this work, we suggest a number of foods chosen for their nutritional values, with virtues for and acting on specific health-related issues in order help you become an informed consumer, one who is able to maintain or improve their well-being.

For each food, you will find:

- its nutritional characteristics/value
- properties
- possible precautions

However, even given the wide-range nutritional values of foods one must be humble and cautious.
Food is without a doubt one of the pillars of our health, but it is not the only one. To keep fit, must also move physically, practice sports, have good mental health, have no emotional conflicts, all the while retaining a life full of interests.
We must therefore adopt an overall healthy lifestyle to enjoy the many benefits of

Healthy Eating!

TABLE OF CONTENTS

TABLE OF CONTENTS

TABLE OF CONTENTS

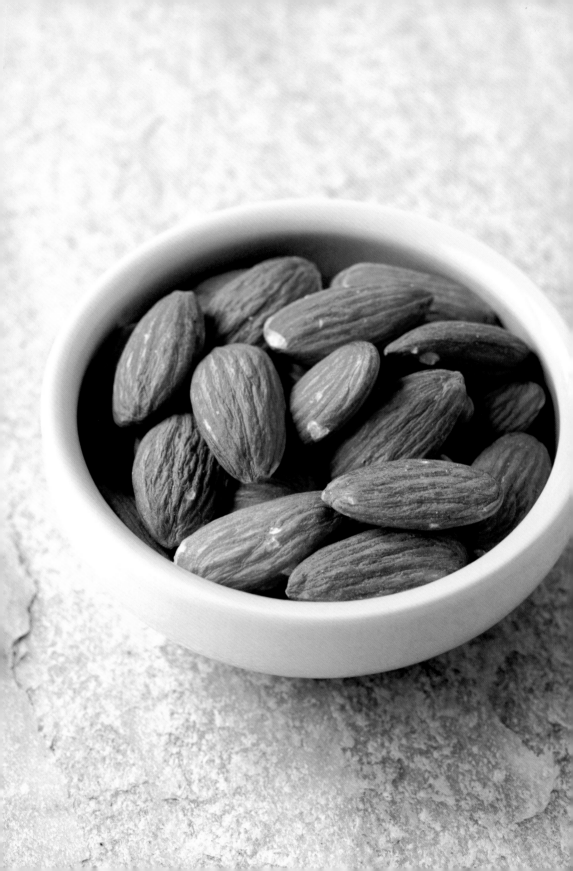

ALMOND

A HIGH CONCENTRATION OF NUTRIENTS.

■ **ACTIVE INGREDIENTS**

An excellent source of vitamin E, almonds also contain
B vitamins, many minerals and trace elements
like magnesium, calcium, potassium, phosphorus and
manganese. A good source of polyunsaturated fatty acids,
almonds are also rich in fiber (15% of their weight) and protein
(About 20% of their weight).

■ **PROPERTIES**

Thanks to the presence of phytosterols, components that
compete with cholesterol in the intestine, almonds
are known to reduce levels of «bad» cholesterol
in the blood, the LDL.
They help with digestion.
They help lower the risk of cardiovascular disease.
Thanks to the antioxidants they contain, they effectively fight
the formation of free radicals.
This is a "mineralizing" type of food.

■ **USE**

Almonds bought especially without their shells - the skin still brown
- or blanched, that is to say without the skin. They can
be whole, sliced, powdered and preserved in a box
tightly closed, away from light and moisture.
They are sometimes salted, roasted or smoked. The nuts should
be renewed every year after the new harvest.

■ **PRECAUTIONS**

Almonds are a very fatty food and should only be eaten in
small quantities by people who are overweight or dieting.

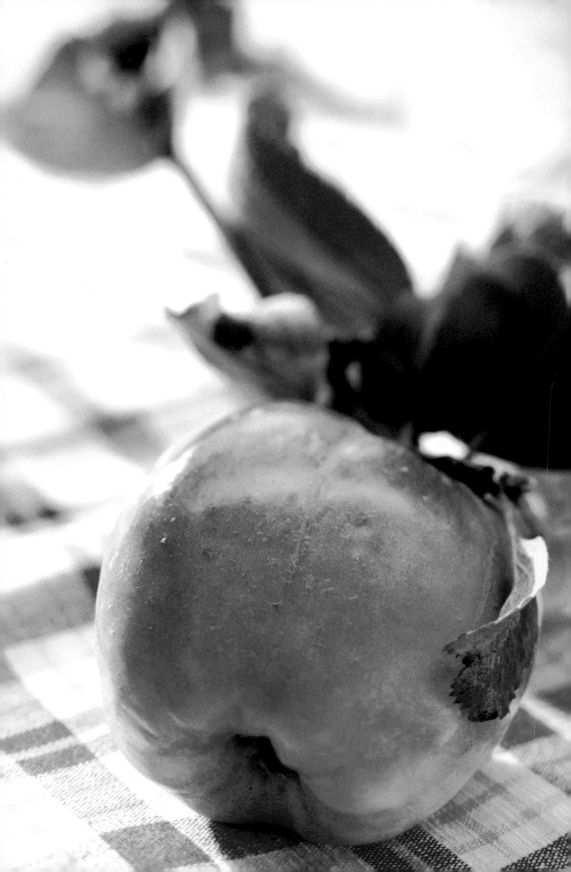

APPLE

THEY REGULATE THE DIGESTIVE PROCESS.

ACTIVE INGREDIENTS

An apple is made-up of about 87% water. Packed full of vitamins A, B and C, it contains malic acid, enzymes, sugars (glucose, fructose and sucrose) and several minerals, such as calcium, manganese, iron, iodine, potassium, sulfur and phosphorus.

PROPERTIES

An apple can help regulate digestion: it is recommended to eat it raw against diarrhea and cooked against constipation. Apples help appease the pain of an ulcer and / or gastritis. It helps lower «bad" cholesterol (LDL) and raise the «good» one (HDL). Packed full of energy, apples help you fight fatigue and stress. They are a diuretic and a purifying agent,promoting elimination, particularly of uric acid.
Apples are one of the few fruits that can be easily consumed at the end of a meal without causing too much fermentation.

PRECAUTIONS

Some people are allergic to apples.

ASPARAGUS

GREAT FOR PURGING.

ACTIVE INGREDIENTS

Rich in antioxidants, the asparagus contains fiber, flavonoids, provitamin A, vitamins B, C, E, K, minerals and trace elements like iron, calcium, copper, phosphorus and manganese.

PROPERTIES

Asparagus is a good diuretic and purging agent that helps eliminate excess water in the body.
It thins the blood, and could be one of the vegetables that act against the formation and proliferation of some cancers.
It helps fight the aging of cells, while promoting intestinal transit.

USE

White asparagus have less waste than the green which, however, remain the tastiest. Choose asparagus with tightly closed compact tips, and keep them just a few days in the crisper of the refrigerator.

PRECAUTIONS

Because it has blood-thinning properties, asparagus should be eaten in moderate quantities if one is taking blood-thinners.

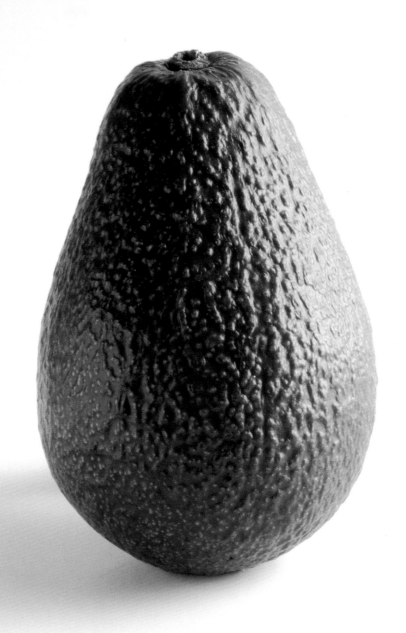

AVOCADO

PROTECTS THE CARDIOVASCULAR SYSTEM.

ACTIVE INGREDIENTS

A food rich in nutrients, the avocado contains proteins, carbohydrates and lipids (20%) for most compounds of monounsaturated fats. It has a good amount of vitamin E, vitamin C and B Group. Rich in fiber, it also contains minerals such as potassium and magnesium.

PROPERTIES

Avocados can reduce levels of «bad» cholesterol in the blood and have antioxidant powers to fight free radicals.
They protect blood vessels; help prevent hardening of the skin.
They help digestion and are beneficial to the prostate.

USE

Buy avocados almost raw (they finish the process of maturing in your fruit basket), with green skin and soft to the the touch.

PRECAUTIONS

Eat less avocados if overweight or during diets as their fat content is high.

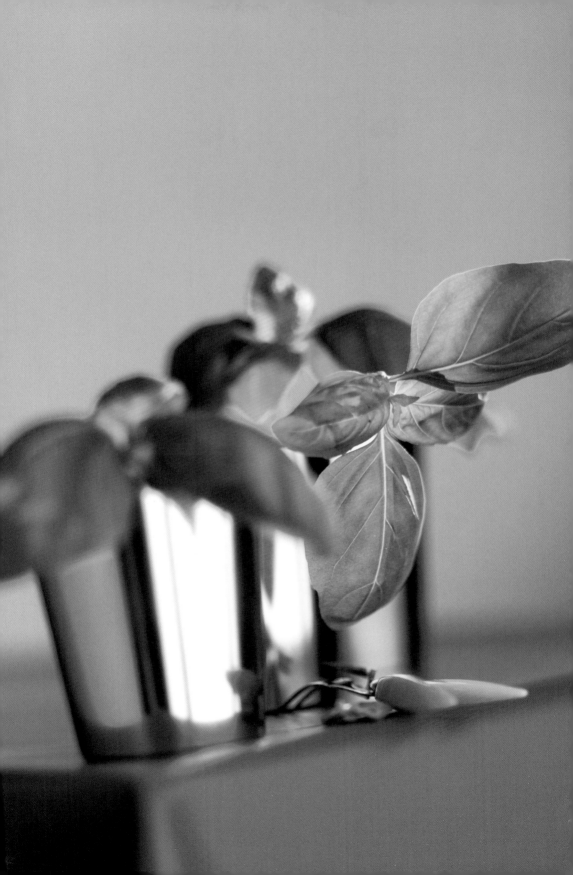

BASIL

PESTO IS NOTHING WITHOUT IT.

ACTIVE INGREDIENTS

Basil contains a linalool and estragol-based essential oil.
The basil plant is rich in camphor.

PROPERTIES

In herbal medicine the plant is traditionally used as a stress-reducer and against stomach aches. It is also known for being tonic, an antispasmodic remedy and an intestinal antiseptic.
Rich in camphor, basil helps clear the respiratory tract.

USE

Basil is a spice mainly used as as accompaniment in the form of fresh leaves or dried leaves. As an infusion, basil has digestive and carminative properties. It is an adrenal energy booster, slightly diuretic and useful in cases of viral fever: infuse a tablespoon of the leaves in one liter of water, boil for 10 minutes, and filter.
Its vapors can be used to clear the airway.

No contraindication.

FOR THE RECORD ...

In ancient times, people inhaled the dried leaves of basil to "clear their minds", but this practice was quite controversial.

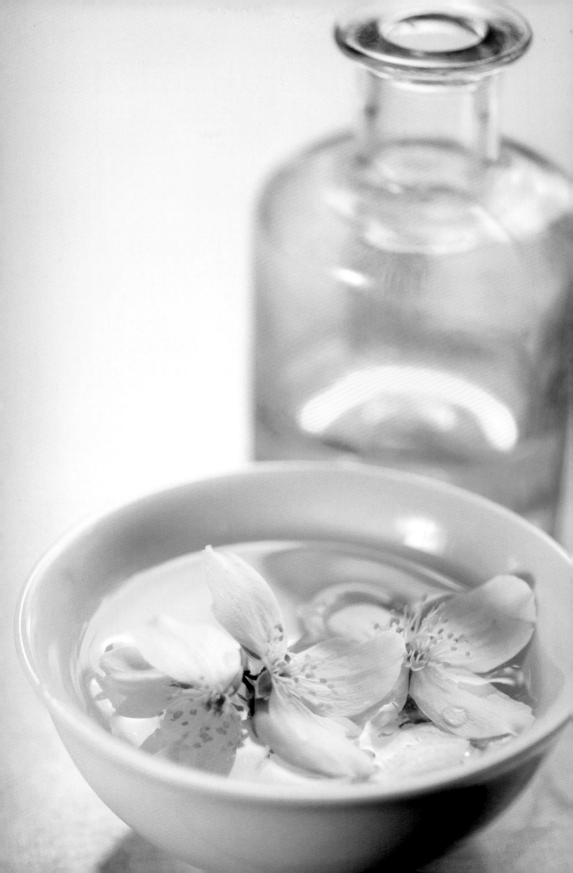

BITTER ORANGE TREE

ACTIVE INGREDIENTS

Various essential oils are extracted from the bitter orange tree leaves and from the precious orange blossoms.

PROPERTIES

The leaves and flowers of the bitter orange are recognized for their sedative and anxiolytic properties. The oil obtained from the seeds of the fruit, rich in antioxidants, have an effect on reducing cholesterol.

USE

Used to flavor dishes and pastries, especially the orange blossom water. The bark is part of the traditional candied fruits. The infusion of dried flowers has stimulating and digestive properties, and promotes sleep.

No contraindication.

FOR THE RECORD...

Orange blossom water, widely used in oriental cuisines, is the residue from the distillation of the essence of orange blossoms.

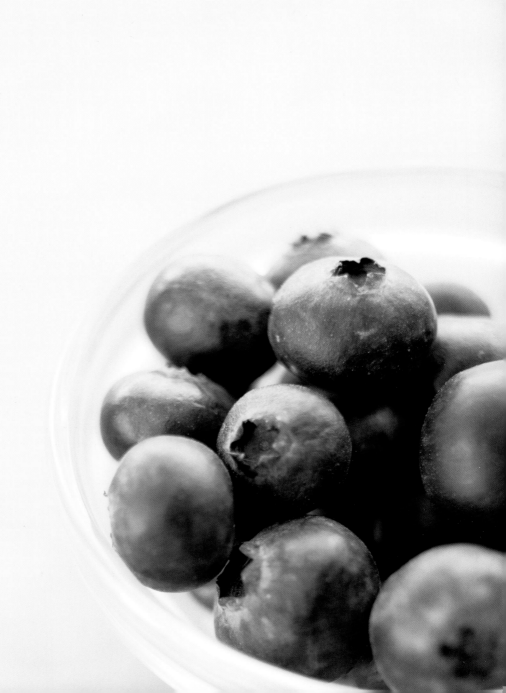

BLUEBERRY

A READY-MADE TREAT.

■ **ACTIVE INGREDIENTS**

Low in calories, blueberries contain vitamins C and E, minerals and trace elements such as potassium, calcium and magnesium, fiber, antioxidants (anthocyanins, the pigments that give the color purple).

■ **PROPERTIES**

Blueberries protect the cardiovascular system.
They stimulate the gall bladder, and are useful against diarrhea.
Being bactericidal, they help in cases of cystitis and protect the urinary tract.
They help prevent intestinal infections and gastrointestinal problems.

■ **USE**

Wild blueberries are harvested by hand. Being fragile, they are sold in local markets, while most of those found in stores are grown.
When ripe, the berries give off a pleasant aroma and have a nice blue color. They stay fresh for about a week in the crisper of the refrigerator, but can also be frozen.

■ **PRECAUTIONS**

Blueberries can cause allergies in people sensitive to their active ingredients.

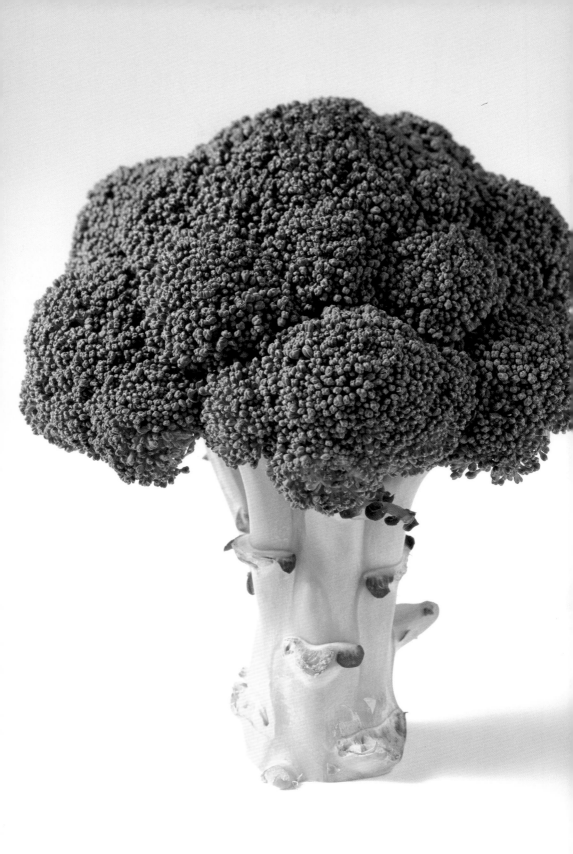

BROCCOLI

PREVENTS SOME CANCERS.

■ ACTIVE INGREDIENTS

This is one of the vegetables rich in vitamin C (when it is raw, it contains more of it than oranges!) as well as beta carotene.
It also contains vitamins E and K, B Group vitamins, minerals and trace elements such as iron, phosphorus, magnesium, potassium.

■ PROPERTIES

Broccoli contains natural antioxidants which help fight effectively against the formation of free radicals responsible for the aging of our cells.
It is among the main foods known to fight against various types of cancers.
Eating Broccoli regularly may help prevent cardio-vascular diseases.
It helps prevent blood from clotting.

■ USE

Broccoli can be eaten most often cooked, but its shouts are also delicious raw, either alone or mixed with other vegetables. If you opt for the raw form, make sure the broccoli is organic or pesticide free.

■ PRECAUTIONS

Because of the presence of vitamin K - a blood thinner- people taking blood thinners should limit their broccoli intake in order not to counter the effects of their medication.

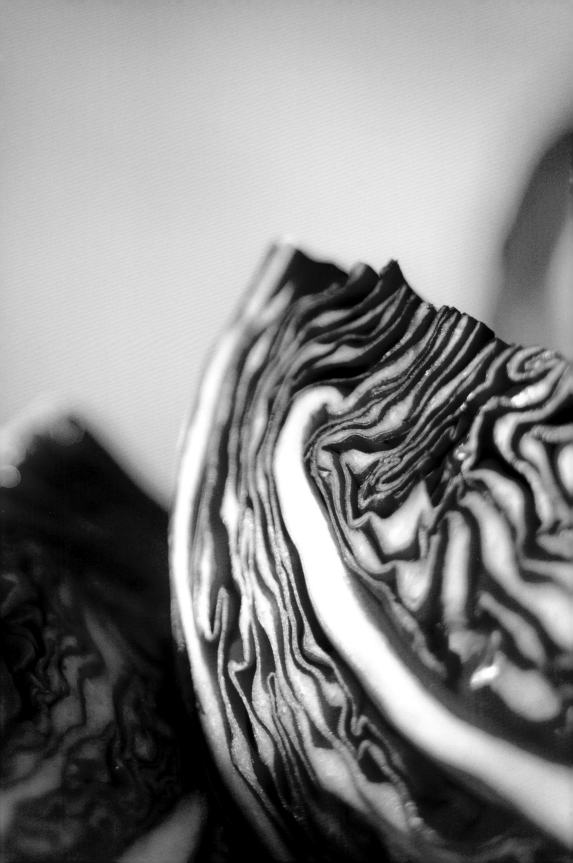

CABBAGE

A GREAT HELP TO YOUR INTESTINAL FUNCTIONS.

ACTIVE INGREDIENTS

Low in calories, cabbages are rich in vitamins A, B, C and K, fiber, flavonoids, minerals and trace elements like iron, sulfur, potassium, calcium, manganese, and magnesium.

PROPERTIES

Cabbage stimulates and facilitates intestinal functions.
Its juice relieves heartburn.
It has an action on the airway and helps breathing.
It is known to calm anxiety.
It has a place among the foods effective in cancer prevention, particularly of the respiratory and digestive systems.
It helps maintain good brain activity and memory.
It helps in weight loss diets.

USE

Choose heavier cabbage flowers with a certain density, with tightly closed leaves and brilliant color. They keep about a week in the crisper of the refrigerator.
Cauliflower should be very white, without the presence of brown spots which would indicate that it is rotting.

PRECAUTIONS

Cooked cabbages are sometimes indigestible. Try to make them more palatable by adding a piece of bread in the water that's cooking them as well as some anise, cumin or a little baking soda. Because of the presence of vitamin K - a blood thinner- people taking blood thinners should limits their cabbage intake in order not to counter the effects of their medication.

.

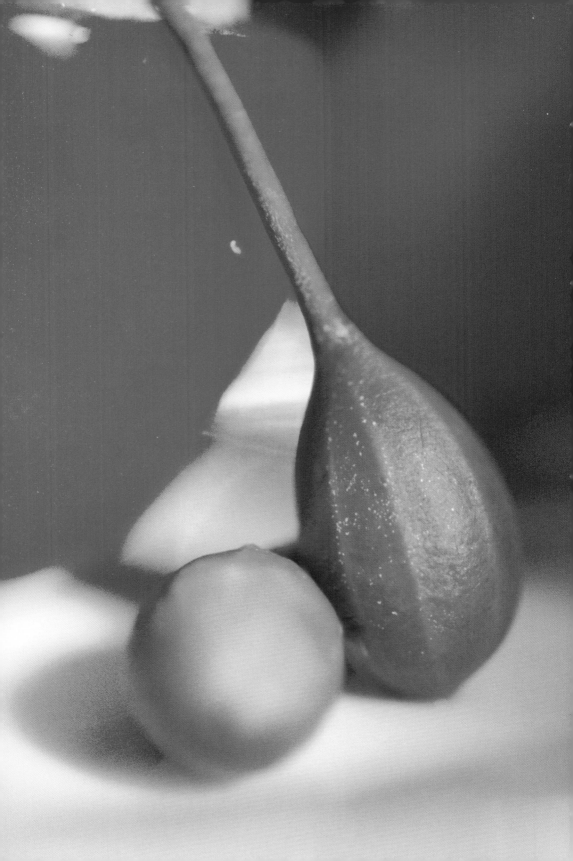

CAPER

A LITTLE BUTTON FOR THE APERITIF.

ACTIVE INGREDIENTS

Capers contain vitamins A and B9 (folic acid) and Vitamin C in relatively high concentration. Recent studies have demonstrated their wealth of trace elements.

PROPERTIES

For years, Mediterranean peoples have used capers as a remedy against scurvy, rheumatism and as a diuretic which is a universally known property. The caper is also known to be a good energy booster and for its digestion helping property.
In Morocco, it is known to cure stomach illnesses.

USE

Capers are perfect to add to cold sauces.

No contraindication

PRECAUTIONS

The Romans were very fond of capers for spicing-up their dishes, probably because they thought they were aphrodisiac, which has not been proven.

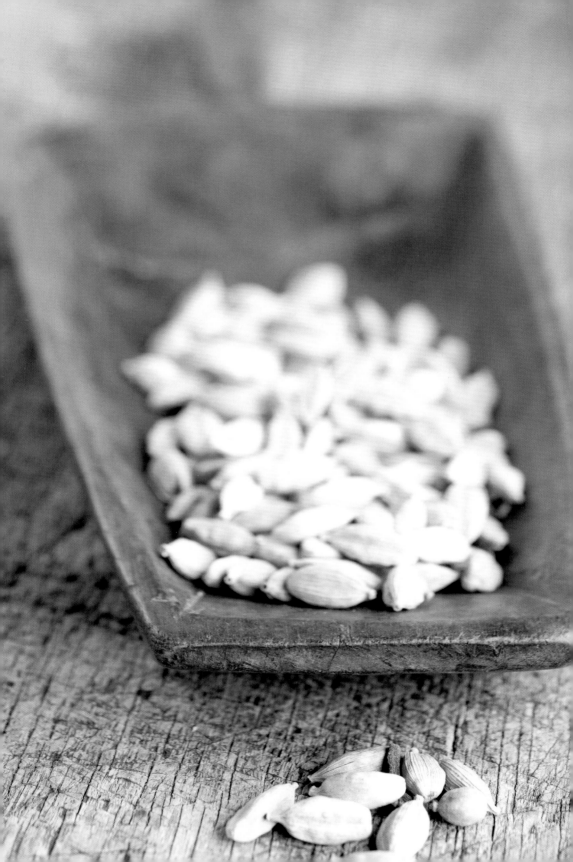

CARDAMOM

A NATURAL TOOTHPASTE.

ACTIVE INGREDIENTS

The essential oil in cardamom, obtained from the distillation of its seeds, is composed mainly of alpha-terpineol and of terpene oxide.

PROPERTIES

Cardamom is used to treat infections of the teeth and gums, to prevent and treat throat problems. It calms stomach aches after a heavy meal, with its antacid properties, and aids digestion. It is also known for its anthelmintic properties.

USE

In seed form, it is used for flavoring dishes or as an essential oil. We can make infusions with the seeds.

PRECAUTIONS

Ask the doctor or pharmacist for use in the form of essential oils.

FOR THE RECORD ...

If you love garlic, but if you wish to keep a fresh breath, you can chew some cardamom seeds after a meal.
It is said that it was what Cleopatra did when Marc- Anthony came to "honor" her.

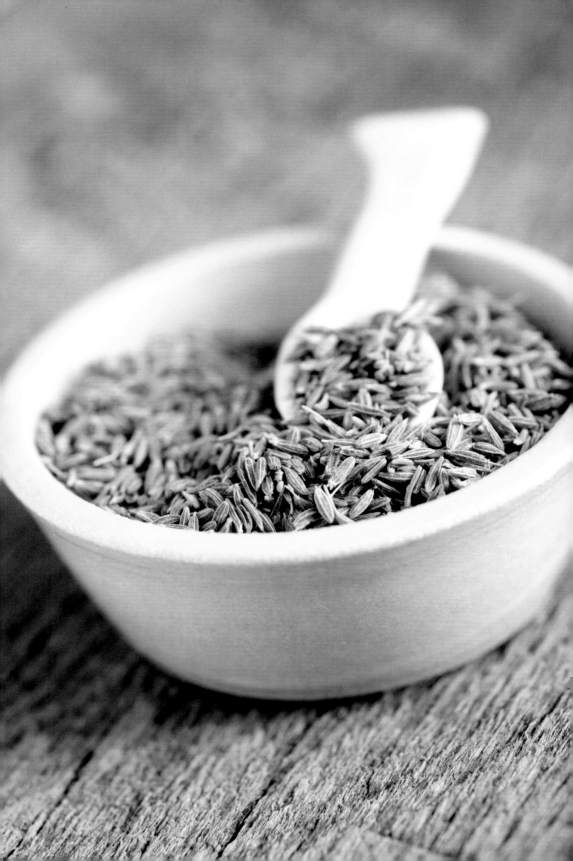

CARAWAY

THE INDIGESTION IS «IN THE CABBAGE."

■ **ACTIVE INGREDIENTS**

Caraway essential oil contains carvone and limonene.

■ **PROPERTIES**

Caraway is a stimulant, an antispasmodic agent and especially a carminative one.
It can treat loss of appetite, stomach cramps (promoting easier digestion in nervous people), flatulence, bloat and intestinal parasites. It relieves respiratory infections.

■ **USE**

The fresh chopped leaves are used to add flavor to dishes;
The seeds are even more aromatic. You can also make tea with the leaves (a pinch per cup after meals).

No contra-indications

■ **FOR THE RECORD ...**

Caraway has no equal in reducing the odorous and noisy effects associated with the consumption of certain foods, especially cabbage. It is therefore recommended to add a few caraway seeds directly into the dishes, or else to chew some at the end of a meal or to have it as a tea.

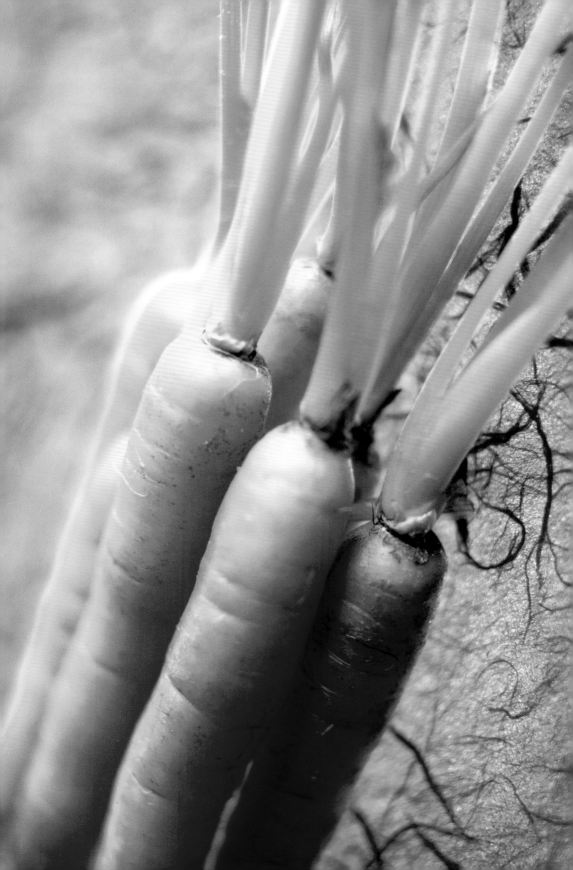

CARROT

THEY PROTECT THE SKIN.

ACTIVE INGREDIENTS

Carrots are particularly rich in beta-carotene which changes in the human body into vitamin A, according to the body's needs. They also contain vitamins E, C (which is lost during cooking), fiber, minerals and trace elements, such as potassium, calcium, phosphorus and magnesium.

PROPERTIES

Carrots help maintain the balance of the body.
They protect the skin and mucous membranes, improve visual acuity, especially night vision.
This vegetable has a favorable effect on lowering the levels of «bad» cholesterol.
It has antioxidant properties that fight free radicals.
It is also said to have the ability to protect against cardiovascular disease, and is also ranked among the foods that can prevent the onset of certain types of cancer.

USE

Available all year, carrots are a root vegetable that is preserved relatively well and quite long in the crisper.

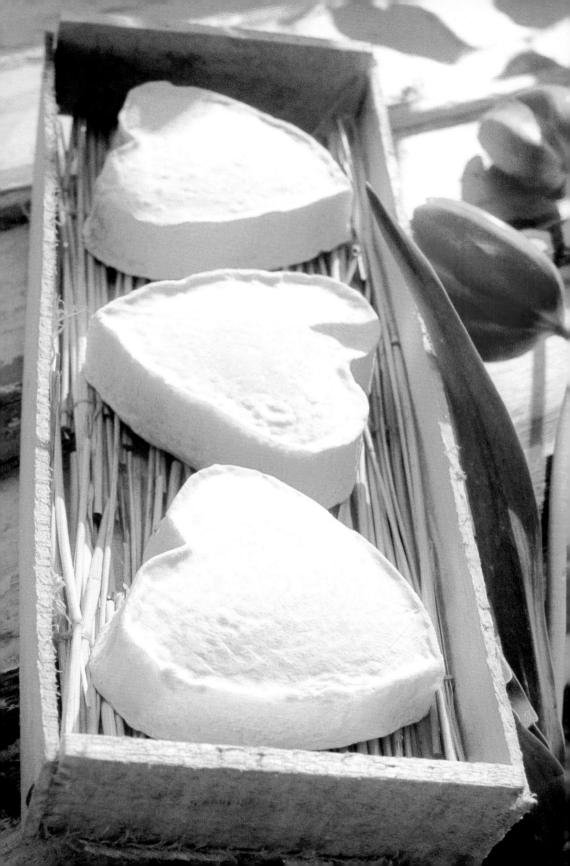

CHEESE

A GREAT SOURCE OF PROTEIN.

■ ACTIVE INGREDIENTS

Cheese contains proteins, vitamins A, D, B and minerals such as calcium (especially Parmesan, Gruyere and Comté), sodium, potassium and phosphorus.
Unfortunately, cheeses are high in fat (the amount varies by product).

■ PROPERTIES

Cheese is a good source of protein.

■ USE

Cheeses are kept in the refrigerator, protected by their original packaging. Their quality depends mainly on the milk used and the production process. In trade, you find: soft, bloomy rind, cooked pressed and veined.

■ PRECAUTIONS

Given the fat, cheese is not suitable if you have a weight problem. In all cases, consumption of cheese should remain moderate. Currently in the USA, too much fatty or processed cheese is consumed on a regular basis.
Reduce the quantities to focus on quality!

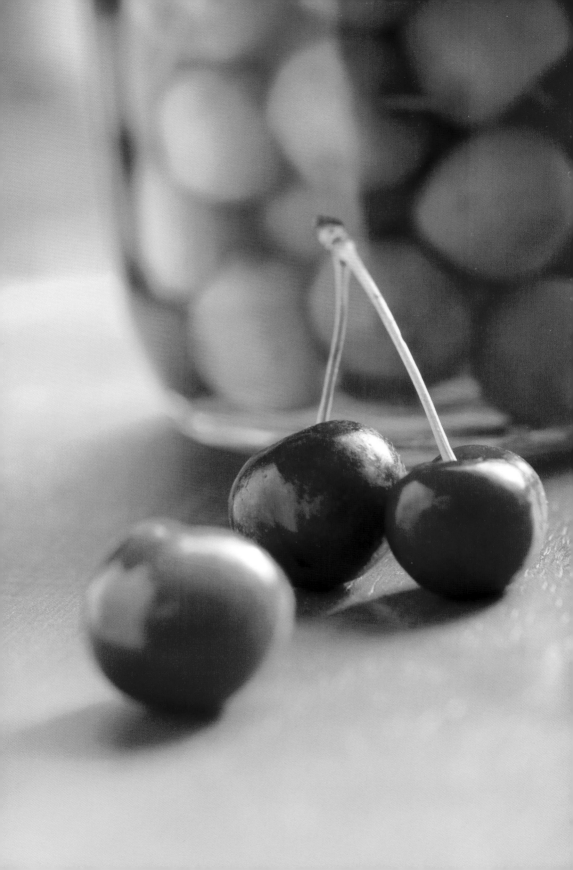

CHERRY

ELIMINATES EXCESS WATER.

ACTIVE INGREDIENTS

Rich in vitamin C (15 g per 100 g) cherries also contain polyphenols (anthocyanins and tannins) provitamin A, vitamin B, E, minerals and trace elements like potassium, calcium, magnesium and sodium. They are among the fruits that contain a significant amount of calories (68 kcal for 100 g).

PROPERTIES

A diuretic, cherries help remove excess water.
They fight against the action of free radicals in the body.
They can help in degenerative disease prevention.

USE

Normally sold in bulk or in small containers, cherries should be juicy, well-colored and shiny, their stems should be green. If cherries have bumps on them they tend to rot more easily.
They should be enjoyed very quickly after purchase (preferably the same day!). They will keep 2-4 days in the crisper.
They can be frozen, preferably after been pitted.

No contraindication

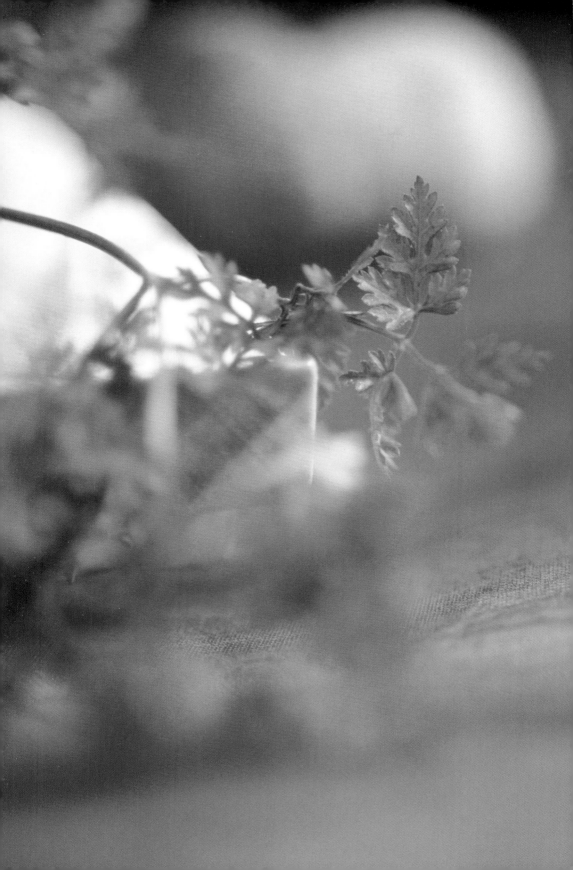

CHERVIL

A BLOOD-PURIFYING GRASS.

ACTIVE INGREDIENTS

Chervil is rich in vitamin C, iron and magnesium is also a good source of carotene.

PROPERTIES

The plant is known for its purifying qualities, that is to say it purifies the blood. It also facilitates digestion and may be used against insect bites (by rubbing the cooling leaves on the skin) and hemorrhoids. It has diuretic virtues.
It is also a good stimulant and expectorant.

USE

The foliage of the chervil can brighten up your recipes.
We also use in brewing to clarify our complexion: Add 2 tablespoons of leaves to 250 ml of water, filter, let cool and drink morning and evening.

PRECAUTIONS

It is recommended to nursing mothers to avoid eating chervil because the plant stops milk secretion.

FOR THE RECORD...

The medicinal properties of chervil have been recognized since the Middle-Ages.
It was used to fight against stomach lazy for example.

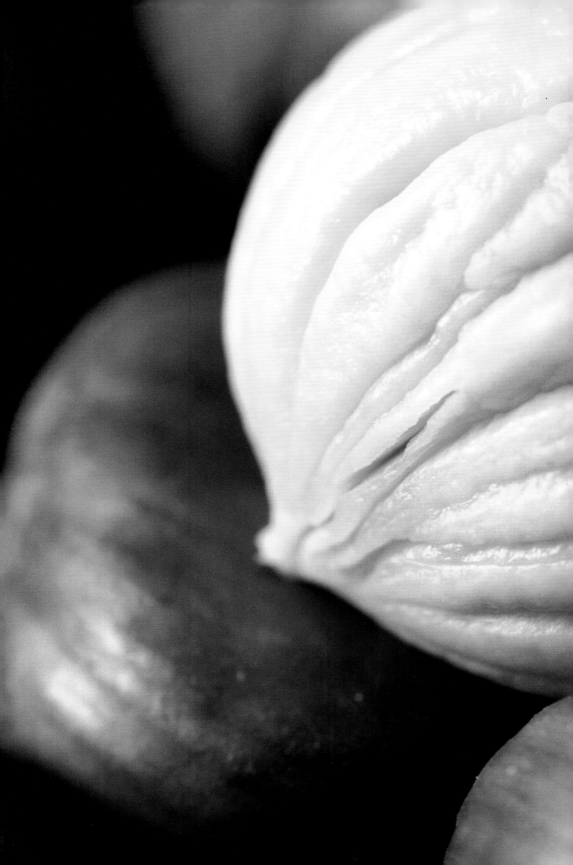

CHESTNUT

YOUR ALLIES AGAINST STRESS.

ACTIVE INGREDIENTS

Very rich in fiber and carbohydrates (mainly starch and 1 / 3 of sucrose), the chestnut has some protein, including lysine which is absent in cereals, and monounsaturated and polyunsaturated fatty acids. It also contains minerals and trace elements.
It contains potassium and magnesium in fairly large amounts but also calcium, iron, manganese, copper, selenium, and vitamins of groups B and C.

PROPERTIES

Chestnuts are packed with energy and recommended for convalescent people, children and the elderly.
Highly mineralized, the chestnut is an ally against stress and fatigue.
Rich in fiber, it promotes digestion.
Chestnuts are suitable for people with celiac disease as they are a gluten-free nut.

PRECAUTIONS

As they contains quite a lot of calories (about 160 kcal), chestnuts should not be eaten in large quantities by people on a diet.
To make them palatable, they must be well cooked.

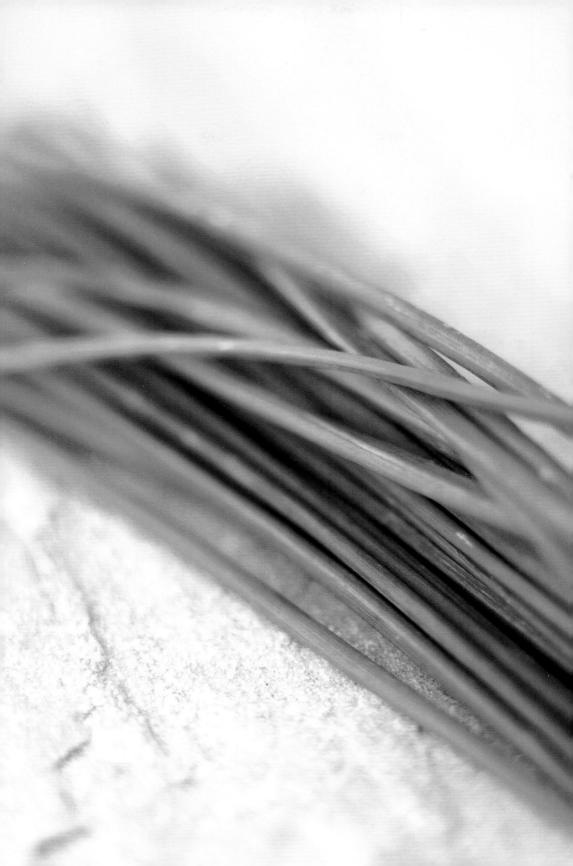

CHIVE

THE ROYAL HERB.

■ **ACTIVE INGREDIENT**

Chive is a good source of vitamin K.

■ **PROPERTIES**

Antioxidants contained in all the herbs reduce damage caused by free radicals. As such, they help to fight against the aging process and diseases which are linked to that process. According to an epidemiological study, the herbal family "allium" would be particularly interesting in the prevention of some cancers of the stomach and the esophagus.
They are also known to have antibacterial and antifungal properties.

■ **USE**

Use fresh herbs (preferably) or lyophilized.

■ **PRECAUTIONS**

Consult a nutritionist if anticoagulant treatment is taken due to the presence of vitamin K.

■ **FOR THE RECORD ...**

Chive has been cultivated in Europe since the early Middle-Ages, as evidenced by a decree of Charlemagne enacting that some species be cultivated in the royal gardens.

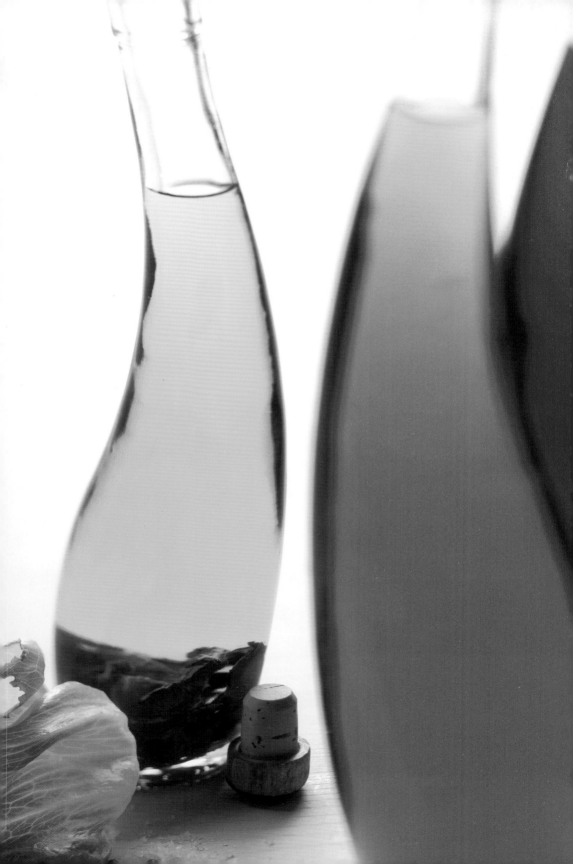

CIDER VINEGAR

THE ELIXIR OF YOUTH.

ACTIVE INGREDIENTS

Cider vinegar is rich in minerals and trace elements such as potassium, phosphorus, iron, fluoride, calcium, magnesium, as well as vitamins A, B and D, enzymes and amino acids

PROPERTIES

Cider vinegar helps to eliminate toxins.
As an antioxidant, it contrasts with cellular ageing.
As a stimulant, it fights fatigue.
It is a bactericide and therefore helps in case of fever or colds.
The regular consumption of cider vinegar helps with the prevention of colds and helps keep good health.
Rich in minerals it helps replenish the loss of minerals causing arthritis and rheumatisms.
It is a sleep aid if taken in the evening.
It fights obesity.
Applied externally, it makes hair shine and diluted in water, it tightens your pores.

USE

Its color resembles that of honey
Its taste is strong but not too strong.
For a cider vinegar to be considered organic, the cider must be derived from organic agriculture. Stating that a vinegar is produced through biological processes is no guarantee that it is an organic vinegar.

No contraindication

49

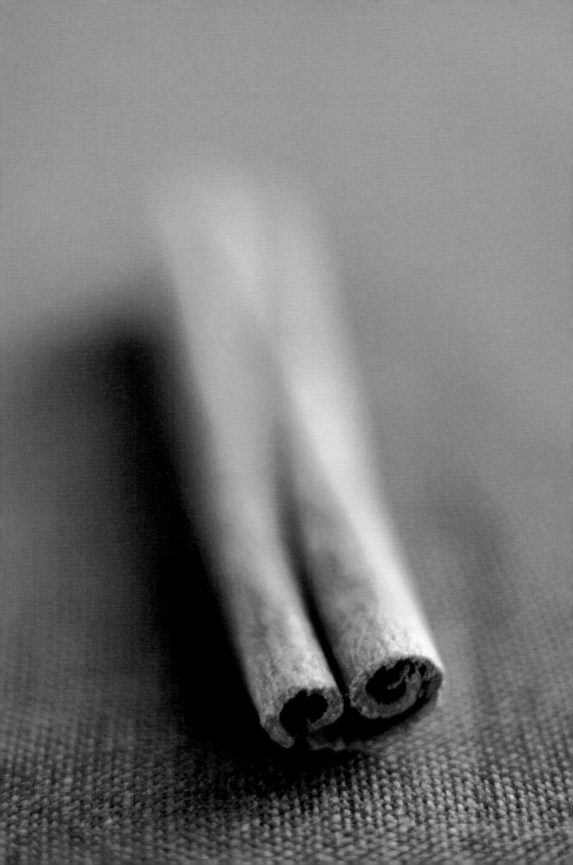

CINNAMON

GOOD TIPS.

■ **ACTIVE INGREDIENTS**

Proanthocyanidins and cinnamaldehyde have strong antioxidant capacities.

■ **PROPERTIES**

Cinnamon protects against oxidative stress and is useful in the fight against inflammatory and allergic reactions. It is deemed to stimulate digestion and help in the elimination of intestinal gas. The presence of compounds with properties related to insulin would make cinnamon a good supplement to fight against diabetes.

■ **USE**

Powdered or as a stick (to be kept in a container sealed to preserve the flavor). In stick form, cinnamon can be cooked for a long time. As a powder, it becomes too bitter after a long cooking process.

■ **PRECAUTIONS**

The essence of cinnamon which is used to flavor some candies, chewing-gums or some toothpastes can sometimes cause a slight irritation in the mouth.

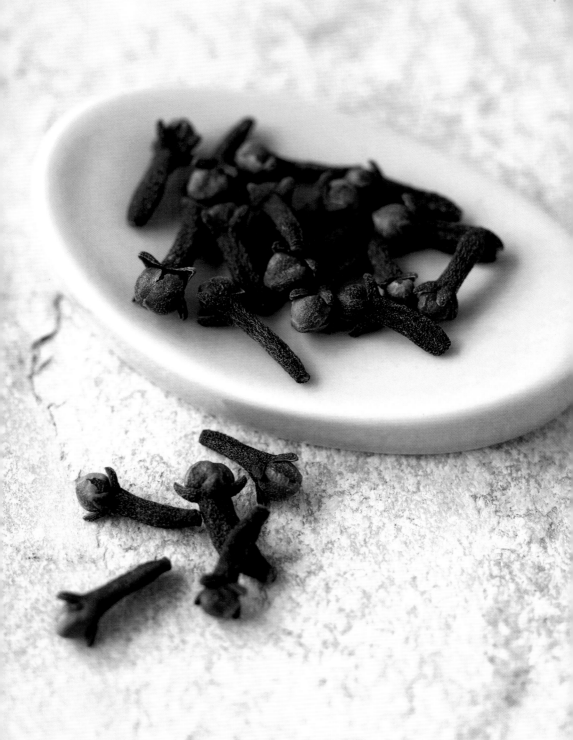

CLOVE

YOUR DENTAL HYGIENE COMPANION.

■ ACTIVE INGREDIENTS

Clove contains significant amounts of essential oils rich in eugenol.

■ PROPERTIES

Eugenol gives clove anti-inflammatory properties as well as antiseptic and antiviral properties and is a powerful gastrointestinal and uterine energy booster, and a local anesthetic.
Eugenol is also considered an anti-cancer component;
It is also considered an aphrodisiac and a memory booster.

■ USE

Clove is used to add flavor to sauces. You can also chew it to freshen the breath and to improve dental infection control.
In aromatherapy, the essential oil of clove is an antibacterial: Use a dose of 30 to 50 drops per day.

No contraindication.

■ FOR THE RECORD ...

Queen Elizabeth II of England wore cloves pinned into an orange to guard against the plague.

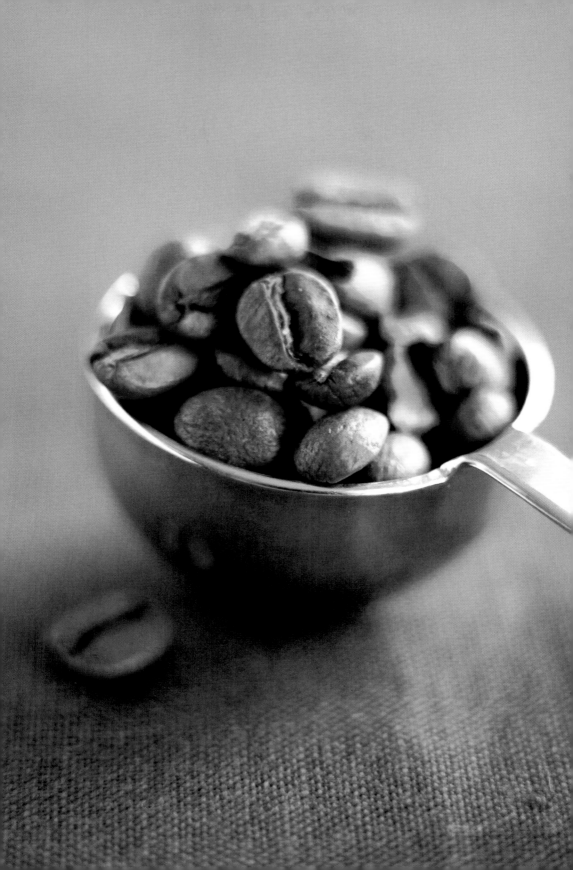

COFFEE

CUPFULS OF VIRTUES

■ **ACTIVE INGREDIENTS**

Caffeine is a stimulant that gets scientists excited about its properties.

■ **PROPERTIES**

A perfect body stimulant, coffee increases vigilance and delays the onset of fatigue during intellectual effort or repetitive tasks. The drink has positive effects on your driving by keeping you alert. Studies have shown that it improves the reflexes related to visual perception. Coffee is also renowned for helping with migraines by provoking the constriction of blood vessels in the brain, caffeine helps decrease the length of migraines. Taken along with acetaminophen or aspirin, it also has a more intense analgesic effect. Apart from caffeine, coffee has a number of vitamins and minerals.
Furthermore it contains phenolic acids, whose antioxidant properties are well known. Recently in the United States, researchers have demonstrated the protective role of coffee against skin cancers.

■ **USE**

All these benefits are increased by moderate consumption; two to three cups per day.

■ **FOR THE RECORD ...**

In the eighth century, a shepherd was intrigued by the behavior of his goats which had grazed the red berries from a bush, and the animals were excited to the point where they danced until dawn. He told his story to the prior of a nearby convent who had the idea of boiling the kernels of these fruits to make a beverage which awakened a special passion in those who drank it.

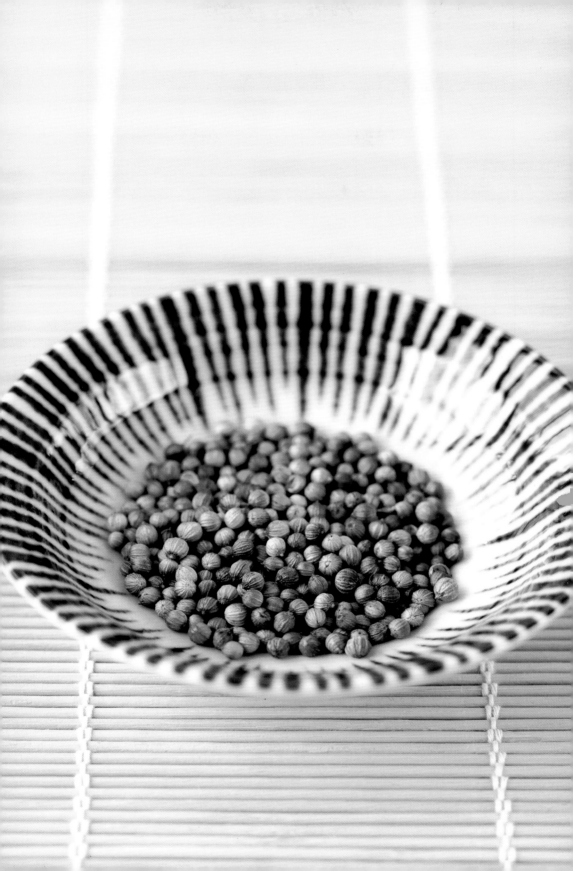

CORIANDER

ON THE RIGHT TRACK IN THE FIGHT AGAINST DIABETES.

■ ACTIVE INGREDIENTS

The leaves as well as the seeds (fruit) contain antioxidants.
The leaves are a source of vitamin K.

■ PROPERTIES

Coriander is an antispasmodic and relieves flatulence and colic. In addition, coriander seeds contain compounds capable of stimulating the secretion of insulin and the increase of glucose presence into these cells; researchers have shown that the addition of coriander seeds to food of diabetic mice led to a decrease in blood glucose, but it remains to be proven in humans.

■ USE

The leaves are a classic in the cuisines of the Middle East.
In the West, we prefer the seeds that go into the composition of curry powder.

■ PRECAUTIONS

The presence of vitamin K requires to take some precautions in case of the blood-thinning treatment.

■ FOR THE RECORD ...

Mmm! The plant releases a fresh smell that is exactly like that of the male bedbug.

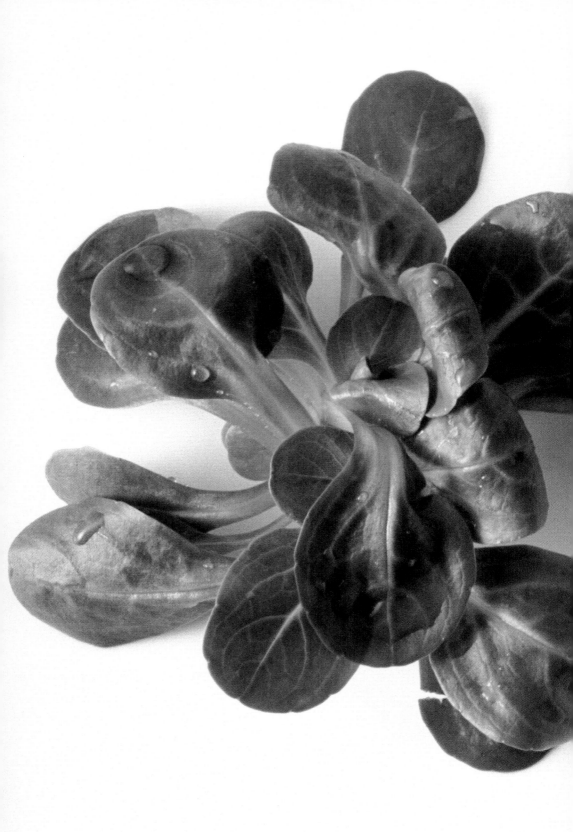

CRESS

STIMULATES METABOLISM.

■ ACTIVE INGREDIENTS

Among the vegetables that are richest in vitamin C, watercress also has provitamin A, vitamin B, E, derivatives of sulfur and many minerals, like iron, calcium, potassium, magnesium, sodium and zinc.

■ PROPERTIES

Watercress stimulates the metabolism.
A natural tonic, it is best suited for children, the elderly and those who are convalescent.
It is mineralizing and helps prevent anemia.
It has an antioxidant, capable of fighting cellular ageing.
It's believed to be part of foods that help prevent cancer.

■ USE

At the market, choose bunches with shiny and firm leaves, not yellowing leaves. Eat it quickly, as the watercress only keeps two to three days in the refrigerator.

■ PRECAUTIONS

Although it is easy to grow along streams, do not pluck it! In the wild, watercress can harbor parasites, as liver flukes, the cause of hepatobiliary diseases.

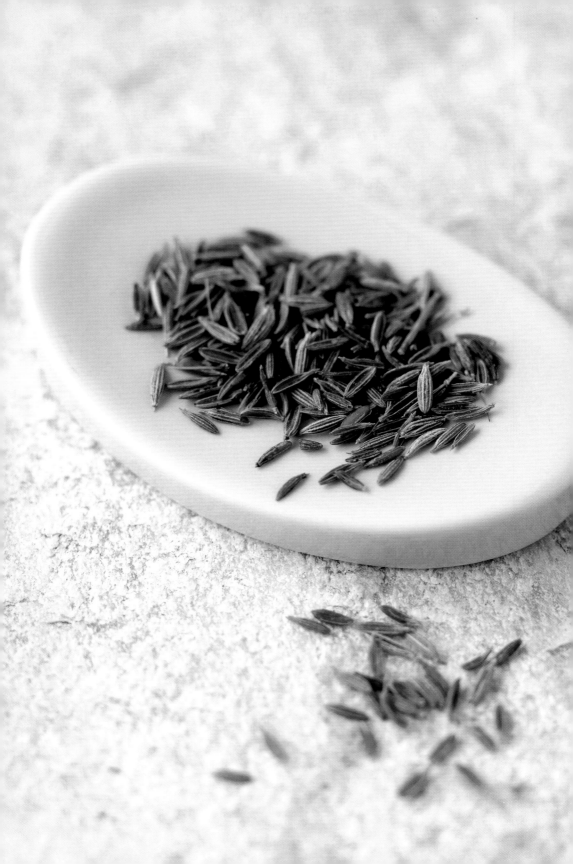

CUMIN

VIRTUES RECOGNIZED FOR MILLENNIA.

■ ACTIVE INGREDIENTS

An essential oil consisting of cuminic aldehyde and polysaccharides.

■ PROPERTIES

Cumin is known to be carminative, diuretic, a digestive, sedative and vermifuge. It has been credited with having many other properties, especially against cancers of the stomach and liver, as well as properties which help protect the cardiovascular system. But these properties remain to be proven scientifically.

■ USE

Use grains or powdered: this is one of the major spices of North African cuisine, where it is called "kamoun". Use it as a tea in cases of abdominal pain or digestive difficulty by taking a half a tablespoon of it ground with a little water. The taste is unique, but the effect is almost immediate.

No known contraindications.

■ FOR THE RECORD ...

The Arabs attribute aphrodisiac qualities to a paste consisting of crushed cumin seeds, pepper and honey.

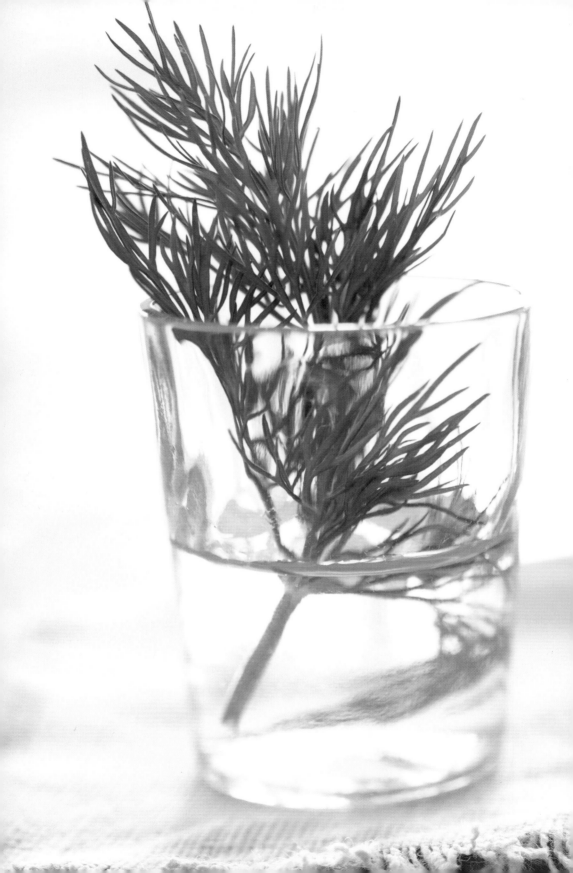

DILL

SEEDS TO CHEW

■ **ACTIVE INGREDIENTS**

The plant is rich in minerals, magnesium, iron, calcium and vitamin C.

■ **PROPERTIES**

Dill has been known to have many medicinal properties, including digestive stimulant properties. Chewing the seeds after meals ensures proper digestion. According to old herbalists' records, dill is also very effective on hiccups.

■ **USE**

The leaves are used fresh or dried for flavoring salads, fish, meats and sauces, seeds are used to flavor liqueurs and jams. Drunk as a tea, dill helps fight indigestion, relieves flatulence and colic, and hiccups.
For a teaspoonful of dill seeds into a bowl of boiling water, strain and drink.

■ **PRECAUTIONS**

The essential oil should be administered in minimal doses. It is not recommended for pregnant women (for its abortive effects) and for people allergic to Umbelliferae.

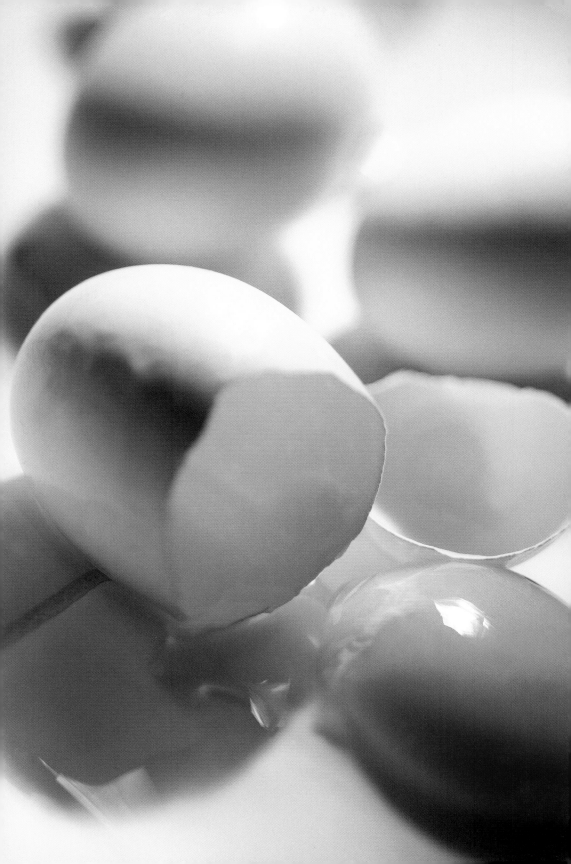

EGG

■ **ACTIVE INGREDIENTS**

Rich in animal protein - 13% of its weight - eggs contain essential amino acids (those that the human body does not produce and has to find in food). Low in calories, it is rich in omega-3 and cholesterol, when it is well assimilated by healthy people. Independently from their shell, eggs contain lots of vitamins A, B, D, E, K, minerals and micronutrients such as iron, phosphorus, magnesium, calcium, selenium, iodine.

■ **PROPERTIES**

Eggs are a very good source of protein.
They contain many nutrients essential to good health maintenance.
When they are well done, they're easily digestible.
They are one of the most complete foods which keep you well nourished.
The presence of antioxidants in eggs helps us fight against cellular aging. Eggs are perfect for children, athletes, seniors, and those recovering from an illness, except if you have an allergy to them,.
All the nutrients make it a food that can fight cancer. Dieting people can have eggs. Its use is recommended to help keep the health of your eyes. It is valuable for maintaining a good memory.

■ **USE**

Eggs will keep until about 25 days after spawning, preferably in the refrigerator. To check if an egg is fresh, simply immerse in a solution of salt water. If it remains in the bottom it's a maximum of 3 days old; if it gets up to half way, it's about 6 days old and if it stands upright with the tip down, it's about ten days old. If it floats entirely, then it has gone bad and should not be eaten.

■ **PRECAUTIONS**

Raw eggs or lightly cooked - used in many creams, meringues or other desserts - should be eaten very fresh, because of the risk of salmonella poisoning.
Eggs are among the most allergenic foods.
Even if the idea is beginning to become controversial, some experts estimate that people with high cholesterol should limit their consumption of eggs, especially of the yolk.

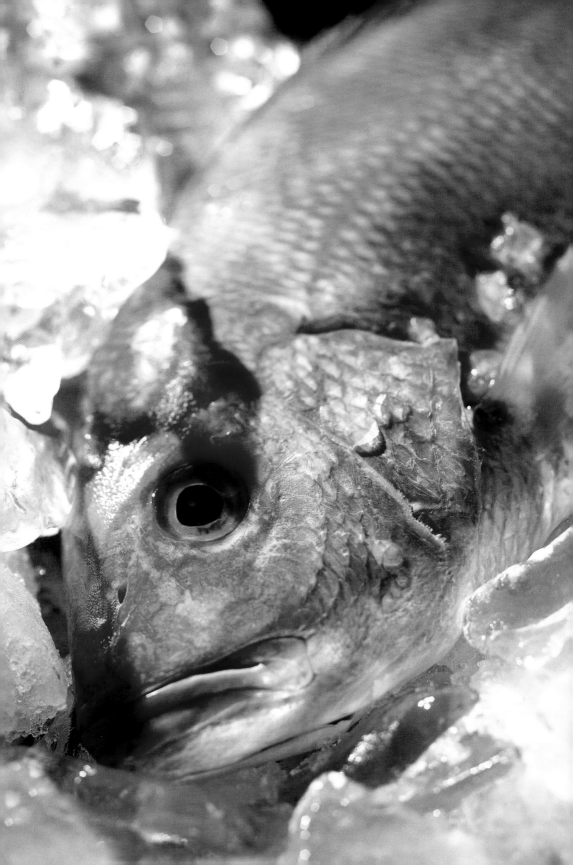

FISH

SUITABLE FOR ALL AGES.

■ ACTIVE INGREDIENTS

Nutrient content in fish depends on the dietary variety of the
fish. In general, fish are rich in protein (almost as much as meat)
and they contain all essential amino acids. Fish is also rich in
vitamin groups A, B, D, minerals and trace elements such as iron,
phosphorus, and magnesium. Depending on the species and the
period of fishing, fish contain more or less important quantities of
fatty acids, including omega-3.
Fatty fish or half-fat fish contain 10 to 15% of their weight in
omega-3.

■ PROPERTIES

Oily fish help prevent cardiovascular disease.
They improve circulation and reduce the risk of thrombosis.
Fish is allowed when you're on a diet.
It invigorates the body and helps in cases of fatigue be it physical
or intellectual.
Highly digestible (more than meat), it is suitable for all ages.

■ USE

Always buy the freshest fish or frozen fish. Fresh fish should be
consumed quickly, while once frozen, it can keep for a few months.

No contraindications

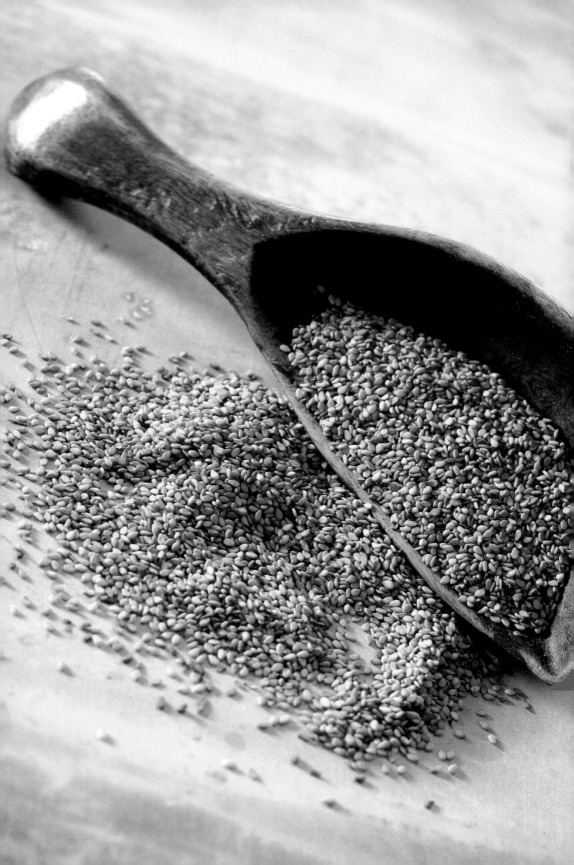

FLAXSEED

A GREAT SOURCE OF OMEGA-3.

ACTIVE INGREDIENTS

Flaxseeds are rich in omega-3, with benefits comparable to those of fish fat. It is imperative to grind them to benefit from their nutrients. It is estimated that a small spoon can fill the daily requirement of omega-3. Flaxseeds also contain fiber and phytoestrogens.

PROPERTIES

Flaxseed may prevent and fight against some cancers.
They help to get through the menopause, and promote intestinal transit.

USE

The whole flaxseeds are not digested by our system, and thus help bowel movements.
They are to be stored in a sealed jar away from moisture.
Once ground, they keep a few days in the refrigerator in a jar away from light. They can also be frozen.

PRECAUTIONS

The oil contained in seeds oxidizes very quickly:
Omega-3 is destroyed by heat.

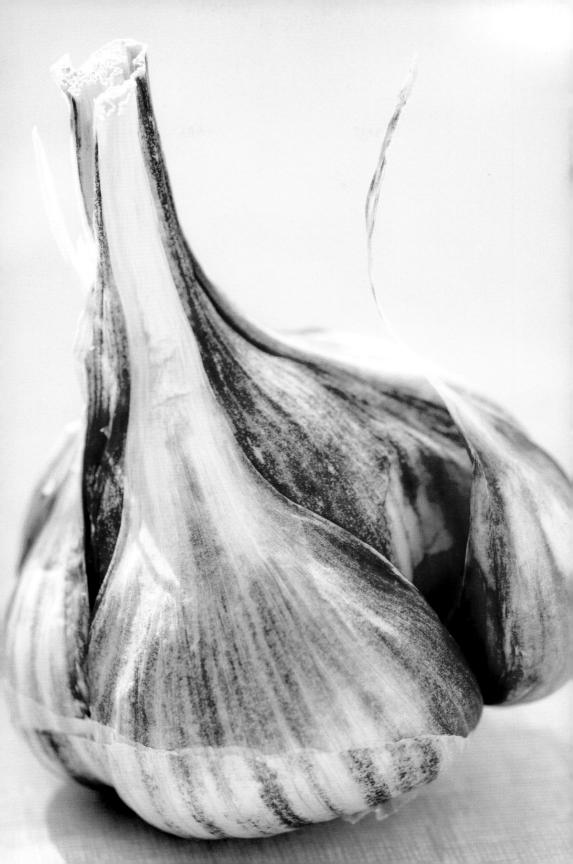

GARLIC

THE FIRST NATURAL ANTIBIOTIC.

ACTIVE INGREDIENTS

Allicin is one of the predominant sulphide components of garlic (responsible for its odor). It is produced during an enzyme reaction when garlic is cut, shredded or crushed.

PROPERTIES

Allicin, which is known to be one of the first natural antibiotics, along with ajoene, another sulphide-based substance, could be involved in the cardio-protector mechanism of garlic, ajoene mainly for its cholesterol reducing properties. Saponins may also play a major part in the regulation of the cardio-vascular system. Fresh garlic also contains antioxydants, flavonoids and tocopherols, all of which are known to potentially help in the prevention of ageing. Garlic is a known antibiotic agent as well as an antiseptic which is particularly efficient in the treatment of mycoses. It is an excellent deworming agent. Garlic, as well as all allecious bulbs (garlic, onion, leek, etc…) are well known cancer-preventing foods : many studies have shown that some types of cancers (colon cancer for example) are practically never seen in populations that use them in their cooking.

USE

Fresh garlic : 1 to 2 cloves (4 to 8g) per day.
Dried garlic : 0.5 to 1g per day.
Garlic extract : 200g to 400g, three times per day.

PRECAUTIONS

In high doses, garlic could cause an irritation of the stomach walls and of the urinary tract. Because of its high vitamin K content, garlic should be ingested moderately before or after surgery.

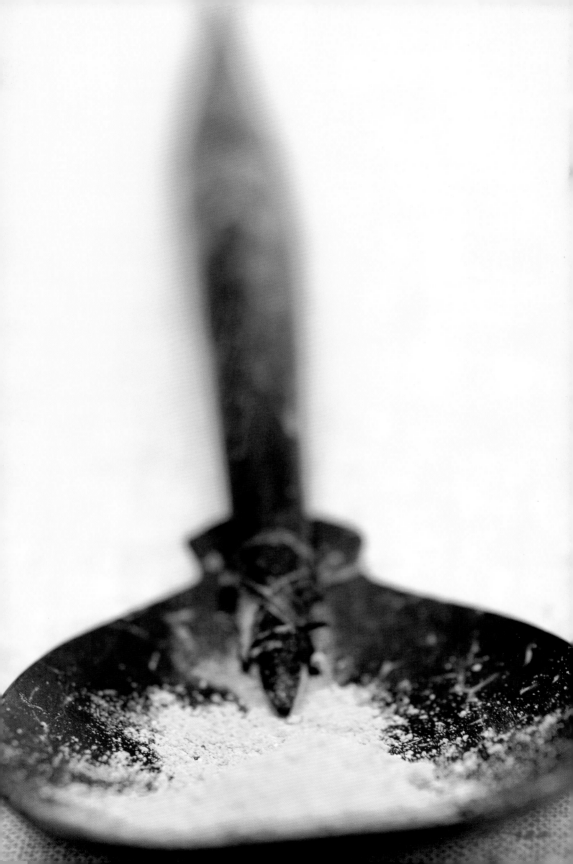

GINGER

ACTIVE INGREDIENTS

Ginger contains about 40 antioxidants, including some that are resistant to heat, thus increasing the antioxidant power of ginger, even cooked.

PROPERTIES

It acts against stomach upset, diarrhea and nausea.
According to Chinese medicine, taken at the first symptoms of the flu, it would avoid breathing tract infections.
Two studies suggest that ginger could relieve pain associated with rheumatoid arthritis. Its wealth of antioxidants confers it an anticancer potential demonstrated in vitro but still to be observed in humans.

USE

Use grated or chopped fresh in stir-fries, candied or caramelized in desserts, dried and ground in breads and pastries.

PRECAUTIONS

It could increase the effects of blood-thinners.

FOR THE RECORD ...

The original gingerbread always contained ginger in order to mask the flavor of the flour, almost always rancid at the time.

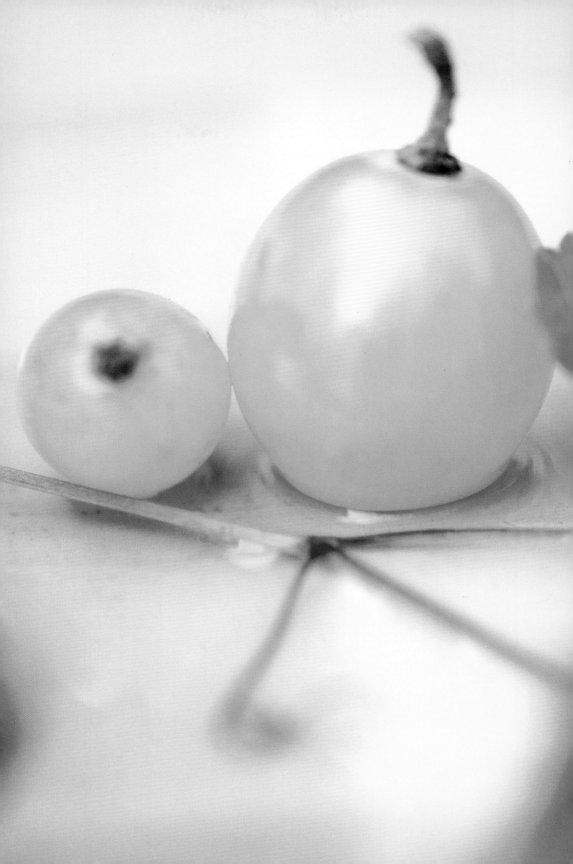

GRAPE

ONE OF THE MOST CONSUMED FRUIT IN THE WORLD.

◼ ACTIVE INGREDIENTS

Rich in vitamins A, B and C, tannins, fiber, minerals and micronutrients such as iron (higher in the red grapes), potassium, magnesium, calcium, phosphorus, and manganese.
Grapes are always eaten ripe.

◼ PROPERTIES

Refreshing, grapes are a good diuretic. Having laxative properties, they promote intestinal transit and are useful against constipation. Rich in nutrients, they are mineralized. They can help improve liver function. Grapes boost energy and are therefore useful in cases of physical fatigue and when one is overworked. They are recommended in cases of gout, arthritis and rheumatism. They fight against the ageing of cells. In large quantities, grapes are recommended in rehab programs as well as for children, the elderly, pregnant and lactating women, people recovering from an illness and students during exam time.

◼ USE

Choose only firm ripe grapes that have a good color. They will keep for several days in the crisper.
Grapes can also be dried, and then kept in a sealed box for several months.

◼ PRECAUTIONS

People with irritable bowel problems should remove the seeds and eventually the skin of grapes.
Avoid consumption of white grapes in the evening because it may keep you awake or disrupt your sleep.

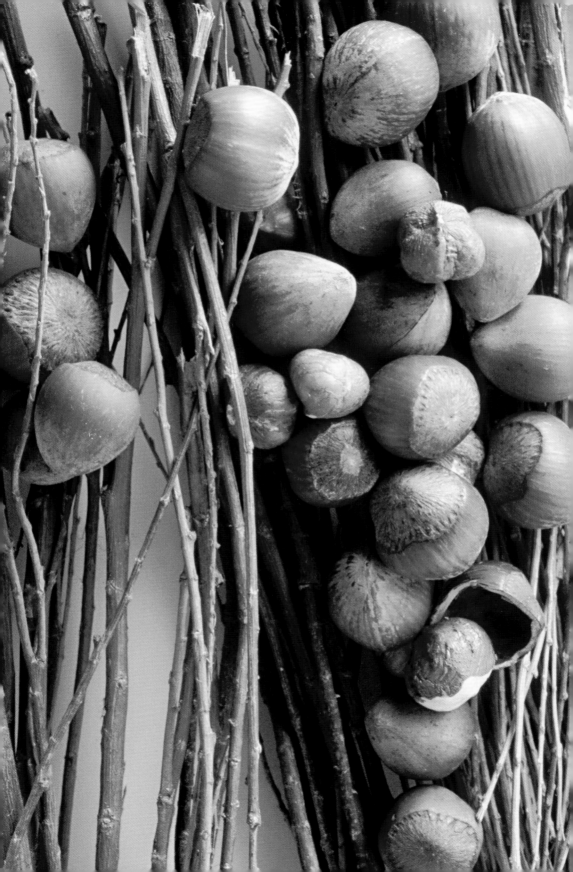

HAZELNUT

A VERY NOURISHING NUT.

ACTIVE INGREDIENTS

Protected by its shell, the nutrients of the hazelnut are numerous. It contains a large amount of vitamin E (three times more than the walnut) and Group B (up to 10 times more than fresh fruits). The hazelnut is an excellent source of «good» fats, because it is mostly unsaturated fatty acids (mostly monounsaturated fatty acids). It also contains fiber, minerals and trace elements, such as potassium, phosphorus, magnesium, iron and zinc.

PROPERTIES

It is beneficial to cardiovascular health because it is believed to have a protective action against the problems related to blood flow.
It reduces levels of «bad» cholesterol.
Its high fiber content helps digestion.
It promotes the proper functioning of the nervous system.

USE

The hazelnut is available fresh at the time of harvest, at about the month of September. Once dried, it can be sold almost throughout the year. The hazelnut is preserved better than walnuts, because its oil becomes rancid less easily.
In trade, it comes with its shell, shelled or powdered. In its shell, it keeps very well away from heat and humidity, while shelled or powdered, it must be stored in airtight containers for a few weeks.

PRECAUTIONS

Because of its high calorie content (about 600 kcal for 100 g of hazelnuts), consumption of the nut must be limited by overweight people.

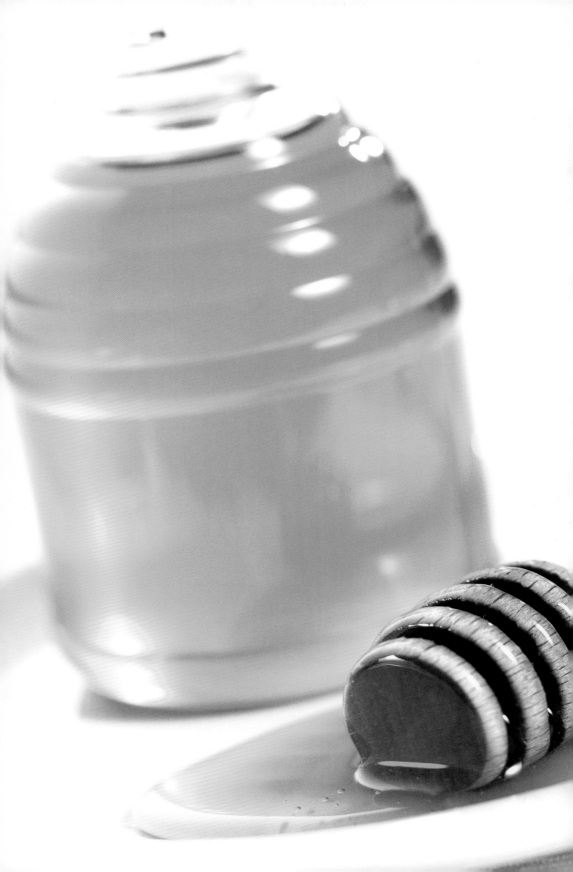

HONEY

THE OLDEST FOOD KNOWN TO HUMAN BEINGS.

ACTIVE INGREDIENTS

Honey is extremely rich in carbohydrates but contains very little fat. It is rich in nutrients such as vitamins A, B, C, D, minerals (iron, potassium, calcium, phosphorus ...) in enzymes, amino acids, and flavonoids.

Much of the qualities of honey come from the plants on which bees foraged (rosemary, lime, chamomile, acacia, thyme, eucalyptus, lavender, etc.)..

PROPERTIES

Honey is a bactericide.

It helps fight against winter diseases including influenza and is helpful for respiratory problems, throat aches and fights coughs.

Packed full of energy, it combats physical and mental fatigue.

It ensures good digestion and helps healing.

If taken at night, it promotes sleep and fights cellular ageing.

USE

If honey is not heated to high temperatures to keep it liquid or soft, even though it loses some of its qualities, it tends to crystallize. Only honeys richest in fructose, such as acacia honey, remain liquid longer.

So buy unheated and organic honey which have kept their nutritional qualities.

No contraindications.

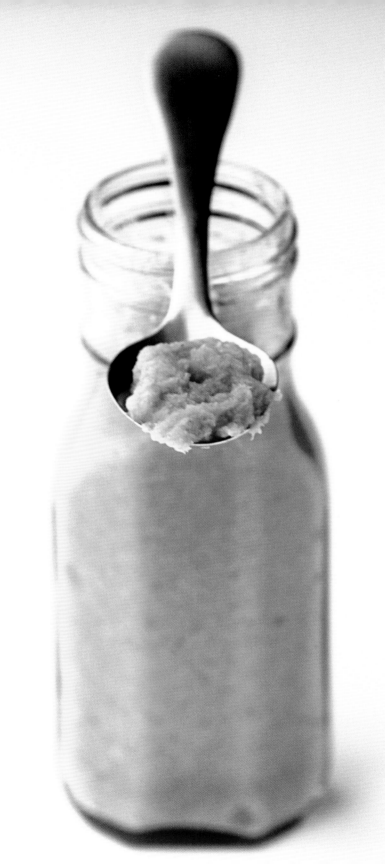

HORSERADISH

A SPICY "PICK-ME-UP".

ACTIVE INGREDIENTS

Raw horseradish is an excellent source of vitamin C. It contains the antibiotic substances, allicin and sinigrin.

PROPERTIES

The plant is a good general stimulant, it has diuretic properties and antibacterial properties, due to its isothiocyanates. According to studies conducted in vitro and on animals, one of its compounds (also contained in wasabi) inhibits the growth of cancer cells. It is still believed that horseradish has platelet-regulating and anti-inflammatory properties.

USE

The root is used as a condiment, in raw form or grated or diced. The leaves can be eaten raw or cooked as other crucifers.

PRECAUTIONS

It should be avoided by pregnant or breastfeeding women, and in cases of hypothyroidism, stomach ulcer or intestinal reflux and kidney problems.

FOR THE RECORD ...

The Alsatian word "meeratisch, «root of the sea» refers to a story which is that horseradish was taken on ships in the Middle Ages to combat scurvy.

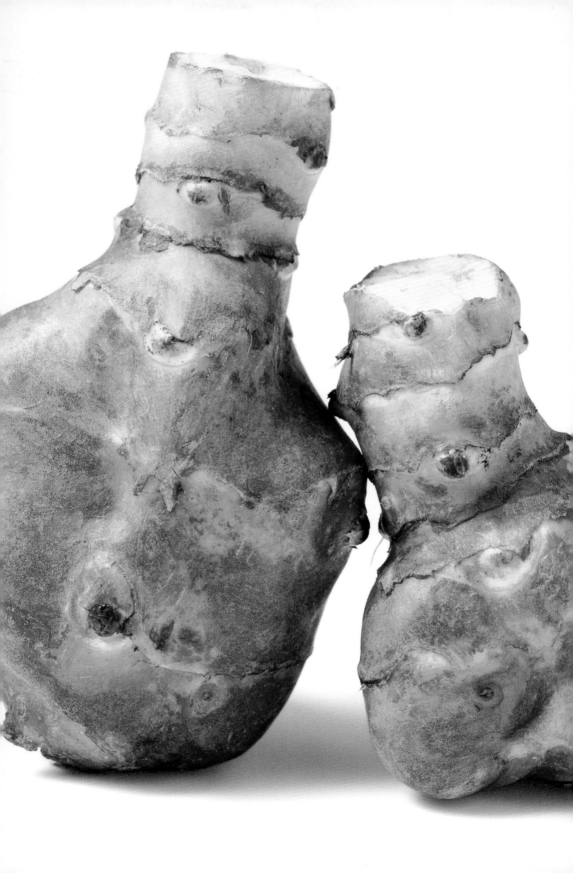

JERUSALEM ARTICHOKE

A SWEET AND DELICATE TASTE.

■ ACTIVE INGREDIENTS

The Jerusalem artichoke is rich in calcium, potassium, magnesium, iron, inulin (a type of sugar), fiber and vitamins A and C.

■ PROPERTIES

A Jerusalem artichoke regulates intestinal functions.
It promotes sleep.
It is recommended in cases of slow digestion.
It helps maintain cholesterol and triglyceride levels.

■ USE

The skin of the artichoke has a tendency to wilt when in contact with air.
It keeps in the crisper of the refrigerator for a few days.
Before using, peel it like a potato or brush it after thoroughly washing it.

No contraindication.

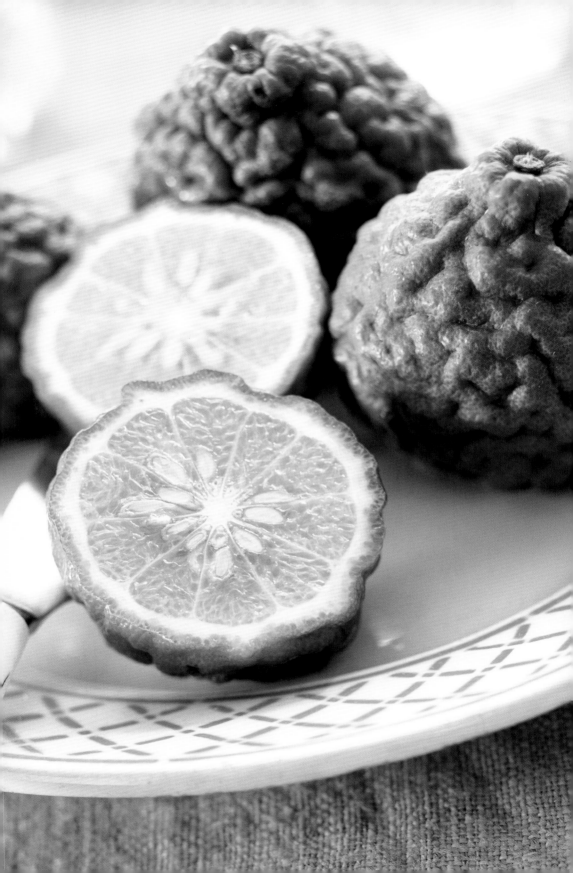

LEMON

RICH IN VITAMIN C.

ACTIVE INGREDIENTS

This fruit, whether it be yellow or green has remarkable assets. Above all, the lemon is among the fruits that contain the largest amount of vitamin C. It also contains vitamins B, E, beta carotene, minerals and trace elements (calcium, iron, magnesium, phosphorus, potassium), flavonoids, citric acid, fiber and essential oil in the zest of the fruit.

PROPERTIES

It stimulates the immune system.
Rich in antioxidants, it fights cellular ageing.
An antiviral, lemons fight and prevent cold-type diseases.
A lemon helps in cases of sore throat.
It helps thin the blood.
It helps fight «bad»cholesterol.
Lemons are believed to be part of foods able to fight cancer.
They help fight fevers and colds.

USE

Choose fruits that are firm to the touch, without soft spots. The skin should not be too hard, but yellow and bright.
With age lemons become darker and duller. Avoid lemons that have green spots, which would be a sign of higher acidity. They keep about ten days at room temperature.

LEMONGRASS

ACTIVE INGREDIENTS

From lemongrass, we can extract an essential oil whose major constituents are citral, geranial, neral and limonene.

PROPERTIES

It has analgesic, anti-inflammatory antispasmodic, expectorant and hypotensive properties. It is a stimulant for the digestive system. Lemongrass has bactericide properties.
It fights fungal infections, particularly athlete's foot.

USE

The fresh stems stripped of their leaves are used in Asian cuisine to flavor curries, meats and soups. The fresh or dried leaves are used to prepare refreshing and digestive infusions (a handful of leaves cut into small pieces in a cup of hot water, filtered).

No contraindication.

FOR THE RECORD ...

Lemongrass blends well with ginger, coconut garlic, shallot and chili pepper.

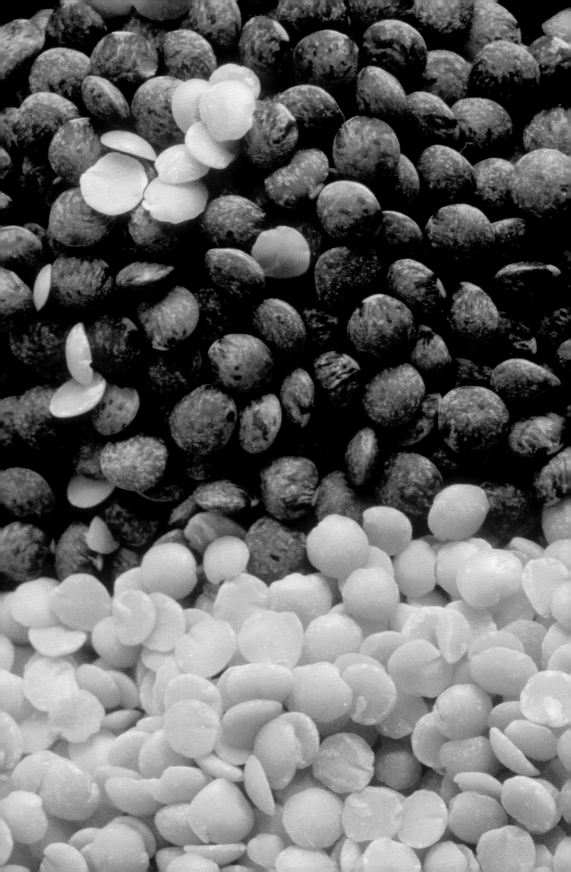

LENTILS

THE POOR MAN'S "MEAT"

ACTIVE INGREDIENTS

Good source of vegetable protein, lentils are very rich in fiber, minerals and trace elements such as phosphorus, iron, copper, manganese, zinc, flavonoids and B group vitamins.
The good news is that lentils are low in fat.

PROPERTIES

Lentils help reduce levels of «bad» cholesterol, and help prevent cardiovascular disease.
They promote digestion.
Thanks to their iron content, they help in cases of anemia.
Lentils help fight cellular ageing.

USE

Lentils can be purchased dried and kept for several months away from light and heat in a sealed box.

PRECAUTIONS

Lentils can cause flatulence in subjects sensitive to their make-up. To avoid this, it is possible to blend lentils, which can break down the fiber content.

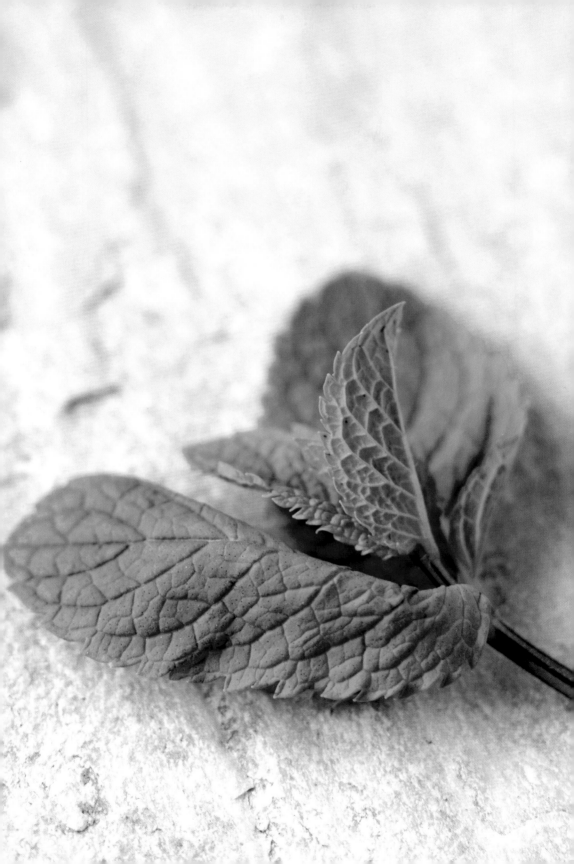

MINT

A GOOD DIGESTIVE.

■ ACTIVE INGREDIENTS

Flavonoids and carotenoids are the main antioxidants in mint. Extracted from mint is an essential oil which is called menthol rich in terpene alcohol.

■ PROPERTIES

Mint is known to aid digestion and fight against spasms, relieve nausea, relieve pain, treat respiratory tract infections, and gastro-enteritis (stomach flu).
It is credited for other lesser-known uses and properties such as being a cardiotonic and a diuretic, used in the treatment of vertigo and food poisoning and kidney stones; however that remains to be scientifically proven

■ USE

Leaves can be eaten fresh, dried or soaked in seasoning or a tea. Associated with fennel, mint is effective in treating digestive disorders such as nausea and flatulence.

■ PRECAUTIONS

Its essential oil is contraindicated in children and pregnant women.

■ FOR THE RECORD ...

Peppermint leaves have been found in Egyptian pyramids dating from the first millennium BC.

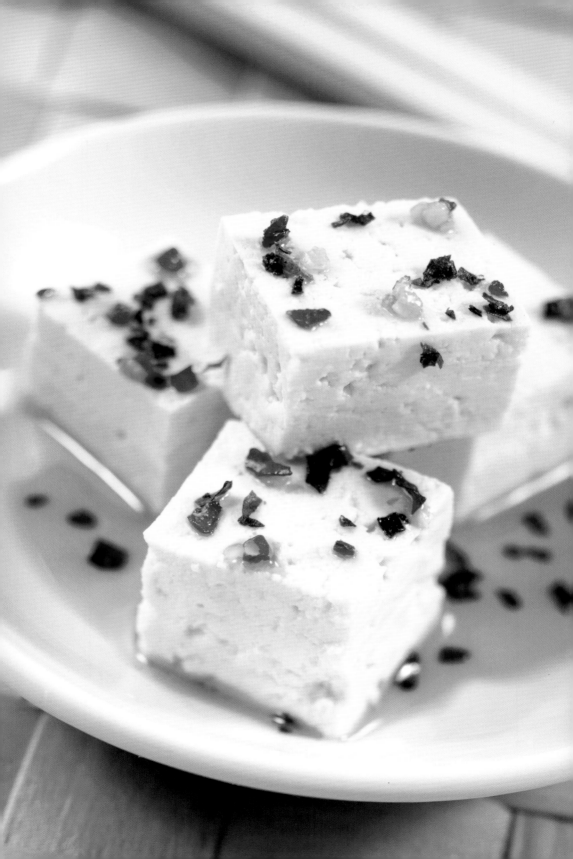

MISO

THE ALTERNATIVE TO TABLE SALT.

ACTIVE INGREDIENTS

Miso is a paste produced by the fermentation of soybeans in water with salt and sometimes a cereal, e.g. rice. It is rich in proteins, enzymes and vitamins of group B, including B12.

PROPERTIES

Miso has a beneficial effect on the blood.
It helps the digestive process and promotes better digestion, and regulates the rate of cholesterol.
It is beneficial to rebuilding the intestinal flora.
It helps fight against the action of free radicals by delaying cellular ageing.

USE

As a brown paste, miso can be bought in specialty stores in the condiment section.
Once opened, it will keep in an airtight container in the refrigerator. It should not be pasteurized, otherwise the seeds are no longer active.

No contraindication.

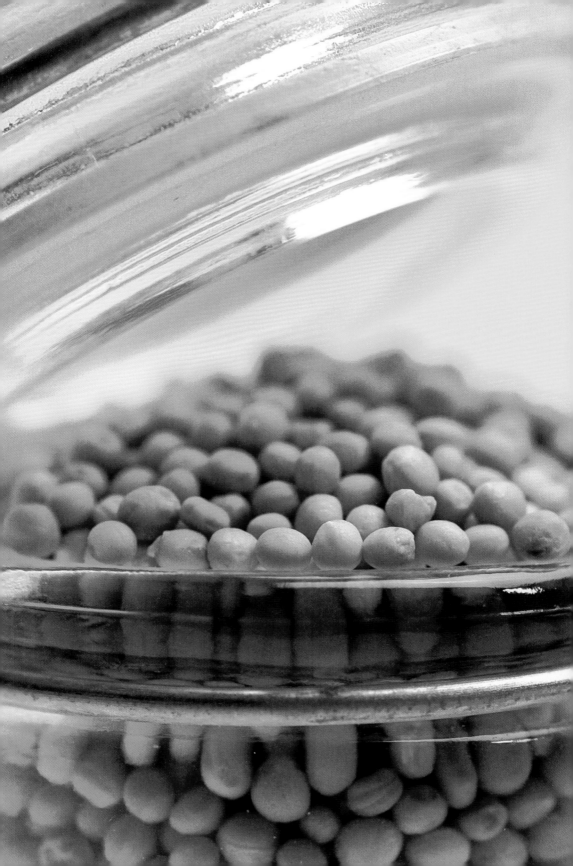

MUSTARD

ACTIVE INGREDIENTS

It has glucosinolates found in all brassicas.
Biologically inactive, these compounds are transformed into isothiocyanates, which are active when food undergoes transformations.

PROPERTIES

According to scientists, some isothiocyanates help limit the development of cancer. Mustard is also a good source of antioxidants, especially the seeds. Carotenoids are mostly interesting for the prevention of all age-related diseases.

USE

As a condiment.

PRECAUTIONS

Mustard leaves contain high amounts of vitamin K. It is therefore advisable for people undergoing blood-thinning treatment to consult a doctor.

FOR THE RECORD ...

Mustard that we use is obtained from black and white mustard seeds and it owes its yellow color to the addition of turmeric.

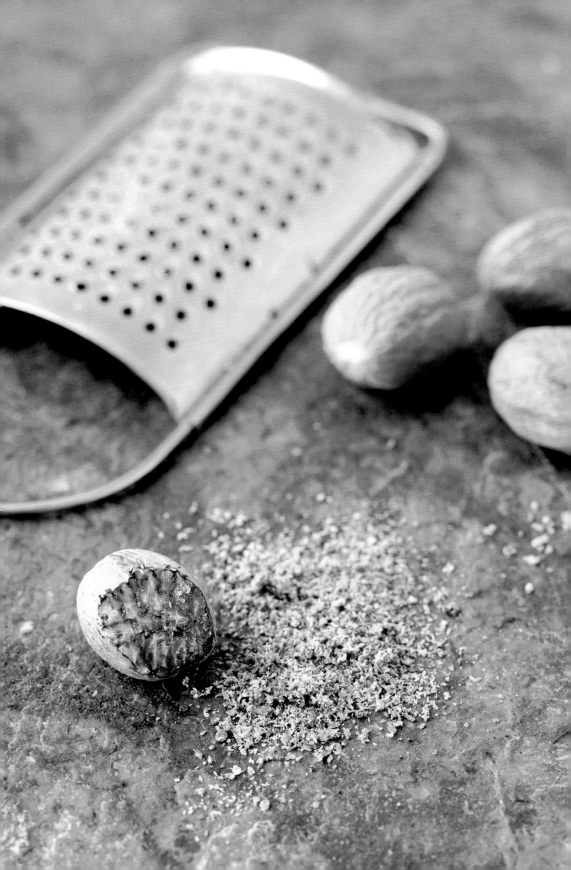

NUTMEG

AN ANTISEPTIC AND A DIGESTIVE.

■ ACTIVE INGREDIENTS

Nutmeg is rich in an essential oil that contains eugenol, considered a powerful tonic.

■ PROPERTIES

The main properties of nutmeg are primarily antirheumatic, digestive, and some say aphrodisiac. It is sometimes used as a general or intestinal antiseptic in digestive disorders or as a stimulant for blood circulation and of the nervous system. It is believed by some to stimulate the flow of blood during menstruation. In oriental medicine, it is used to treat bronchial problems and against rheumatism.

■ USE

It is used shredded on meat, soups,etc..
And in France it is very popular in the gratin (potatoes, zucchini ..).
Medicinal use: in the form of essential oil as a body tonic.

■ PRECAUTIONS

The essential oil of nutmeg should not be used on children: the presence of myristicin, toxic in high doses, including the nervous system, makes it dangerous.

■ FOR THE RECORD ...

In India, nutmeg is used to treat headaches, insomnia and incontinence.

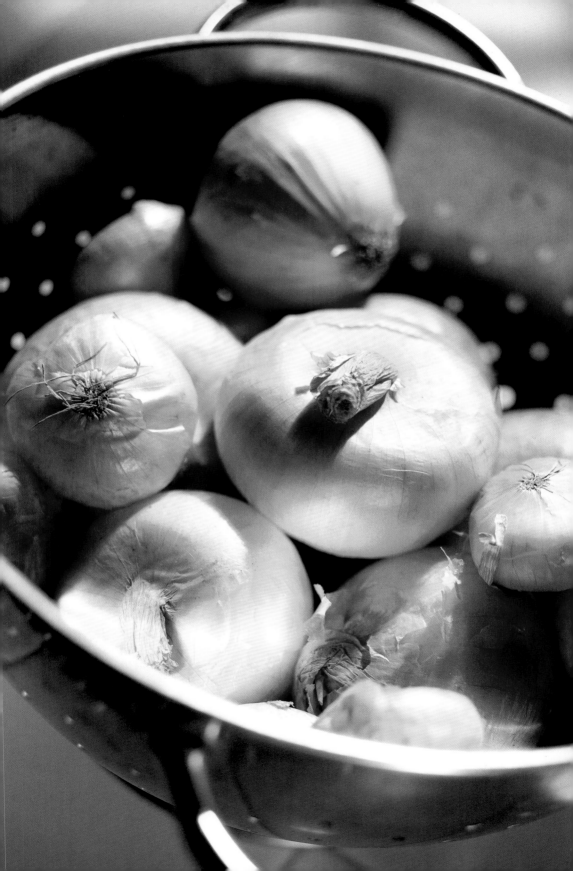

ONION

A PLUS FOR THE HEART.

■ **ACTIVE INGREDIENTS**

The plant is rich in flavonoids and anthocyanins, which are powerful antioxidants. Overpeeling it not recommended as much of it is lost.

■ **PROPERTIES**

Many studies confirm the extraordinary power of onion: it is recognized as a particularly strong antioxidant and is particularly rich in quercetin, a "protector" which is very effective in preventing cancers of the digestive tract: epidemiological studies make a link between onion consumption and reduced incidences of these cancers. The onion is also beneficial for the cardiovascular system. Finally it is known for its digestive and anti-inflammatory virtues.

■ **USE**

Can be eaten raw or cooked, or pickled.

No contraindication.

■ **FOR THE RECORD ...**

A highly volatile molecule is responsible for the tears that usually accompany the peeling of onions: it is the propanthial-S-oxide.

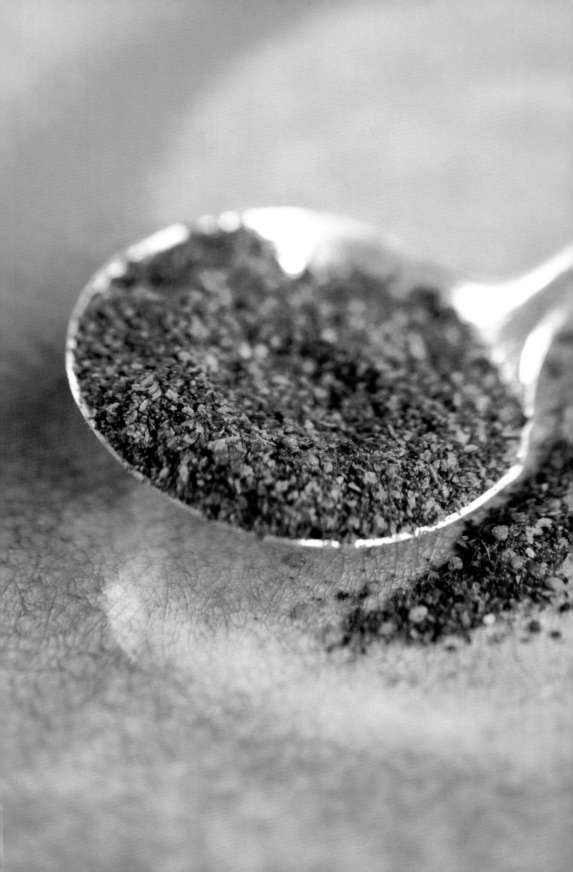

PAPRIKA

COUNTLESS VIRTUES.

■ ACTIVE INGREDIENTS

Its virtues are mostly due to capsaicin, an alkaloid that produces a burning sensation in the mouth (without being a chemical burning).

■ PROPERTIES

What a slew of virtues paprika is known to have! Decongestant, expectorant, heating and calming, it reduces the risk of heart disease and is a good tonic. Consumed fresh, it promotes the digestion of starch, it is stimulating, stomachic and rubefacient
(reddens the skin). Capsaicin stimulates the production of two hormones, adrenaline and noradrenaline, which allow us to burn sugars and fat reserves. The use of paprika may be recommended when dieting.

■ USE

Cool, dry, whole, crushed, ground or canned.

■ PRECAUTION

In large quantities, capsaicin can be a deadly poison:
Symptoms of overdose are difficulty breathing, cyanosis and convulsions.

■ FOR THE RECORD ...

The use of paprika in Hungary is known to have spread because the majority of the population could not buy expensive spices, like pepper. Paprika would have been adopted by all segments of the population, to become one of the bases of Hungarian cuisine.

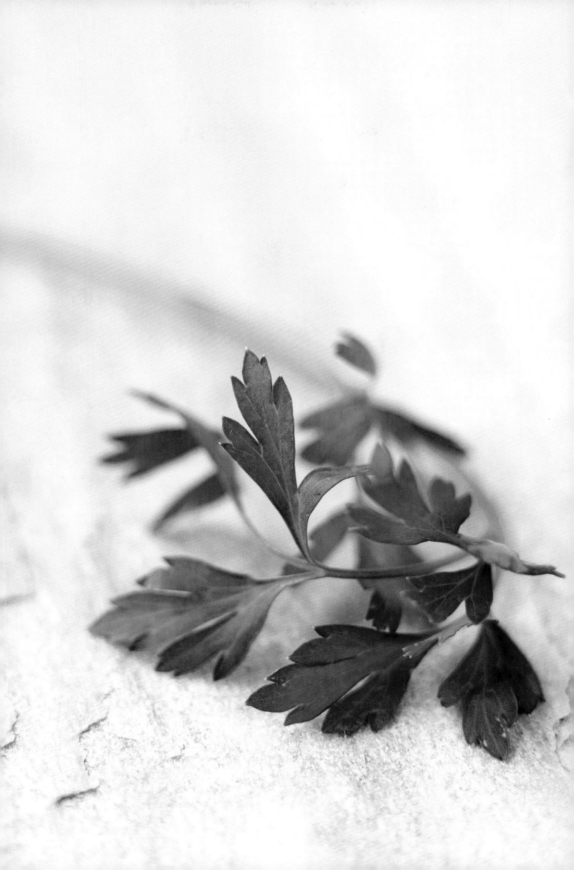

PARSLEY

THE BREATH FRESHENER.

■ ACTIVE INGREDIENTS

Parsley contains powerful antioxidants, including apigenin, Lutein and beta-carotene.

■ PROPERTIES

In addition to its antioxidant property, apigenin could allow parsley to help regulate blood sugar. Researchers administered extracts of parsley to diabetic rats for several days; they noticed a decrease in blood sugar. However, no study has evaluated these effects on humans. Consumed in large quantities, parsley is interesting from a nutritional standpoint, especially for its vitamin C content. It is a tonic and a stimulant.

■ USE

We can use the leaves fresh or dried, as seasoning or garnish, as well as a tea brewed for its sedative properties.

■ FOR THE RECORD ...

By capturing some sulfur compounds formed in the mouth and in the intestine, fresh parsley could fight bad breath.

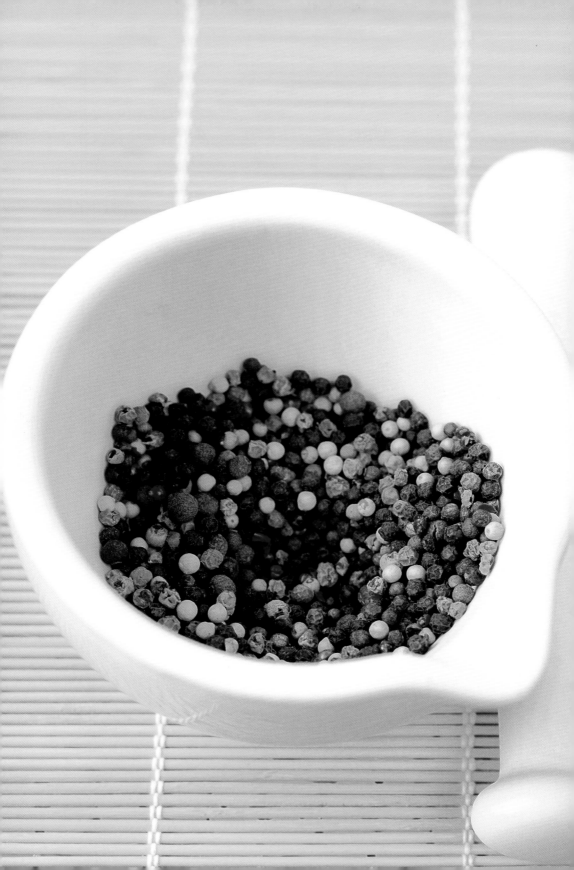

PEPPER

HELPS CUTS HEAL BETTER.

■ **ACTIVE INGREDIENTS**

> The ripe fruits contain an essential oil rich in terpenes with warming, stimulating, analgesic and aphrodisiac properties.

■ **PROPERTIES**

> The stimulant properties of pepper on the digestive secretions are well known, but beware: it can become irritating if consumed in excessive quantities. It's known to have purgative properties and could also act on fats and sugar. It is sometimes used to quickly heal minor cuts.

■ **USE**

> Seasoning in the form of beans or ground. Exists in the form of essential oil.
>
> No contraindication.

■ **FOR THE RECORD ...**

> The pepper flavor is due to spicy piperidine.

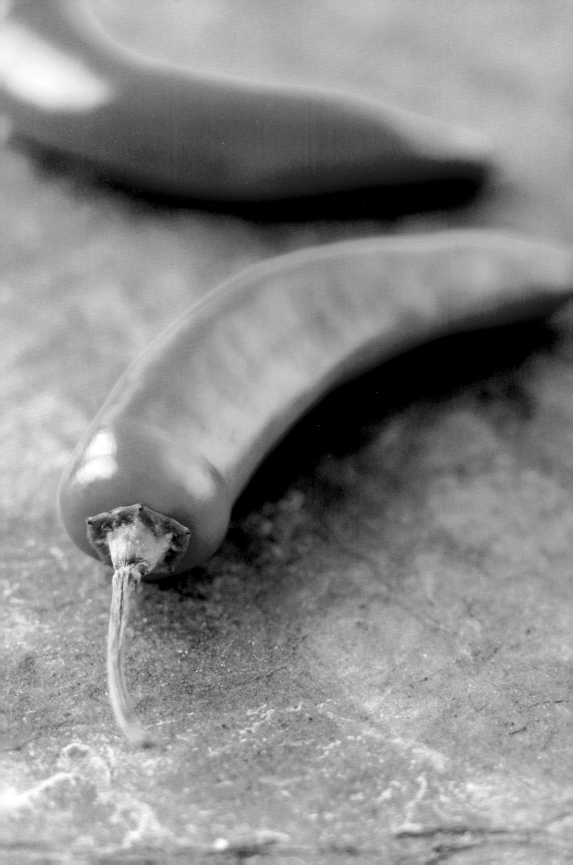

PIMENTO

ACTIVE INGREDIENTS

All peppers contain capsaicinoids responsible for their pungency. They are very rich in vitamins (beta-carotene and vitamin C) which are good sources of antioxidants.

PROPERTIES

Capsaicin may help with weight loss in obese people and have an action on the «bad» cholesterol.
Recent studies have shown its benefits to diabetics; researchers have indeed found that the amount of insulin necessary to lower blood sugar after a meal is reduced if the meal contains chili pepper.

USE

The pepper is used fresh, dried or powdered for spicing a dish.

PRECAUTIONS

The pepper may induce gastro-esophageal reflux, and its excessive consumption is associated with stomach cancer. It
is not recommended for patients suffering from hemorrhoids.

FOR THE RECORD ...

The chili can be used to produce a natural insecticide: crush finely 300 g pepper (dried or fresh), mix with 2 liters of water, shake well to obtain a homogeneous mixture and filter.
Add to this a solution of soapy water.
Spray directly on the leaves of plants.

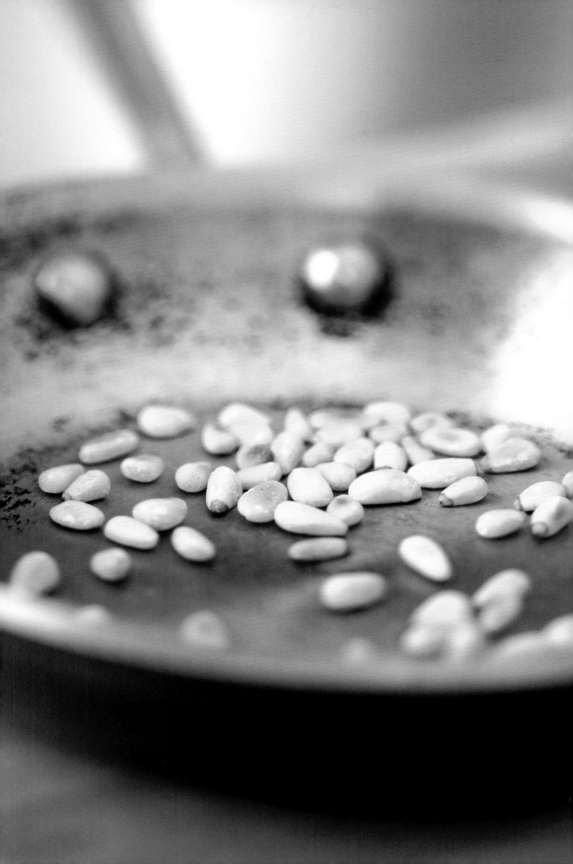

PINE NUT (GABLE)

THE GOOD SEED FOR THE HEART.

ACTIVE INGREDIENTS

Phytosterols have a protective effect against cardiovascular disease.

PROPERTIES

The pine nut is a good source of vegetable protein.
Moreover, it contains mostly good fats, that is to say, polyunsaturated fatty acids. Phytosterols, naturally present in pine nuts, are also useful to cardiovascular health.

USE

As an accompaniment to salads, soups, vegetables or fruits.
Do not keep them too long and only buy small quantities at a time because they quickly lose their flavor.
We can draw an edible oil from pine nuts.

PRECAUTIONS

Beware if you are allergic to tree nuts and seed oils.neux.

FOR THE RECORD ...

All species of pines produce nuts, but they are generally too small to be interesting to human consumption.
The gable sold in stores belongs to the stone pine variety of trees.

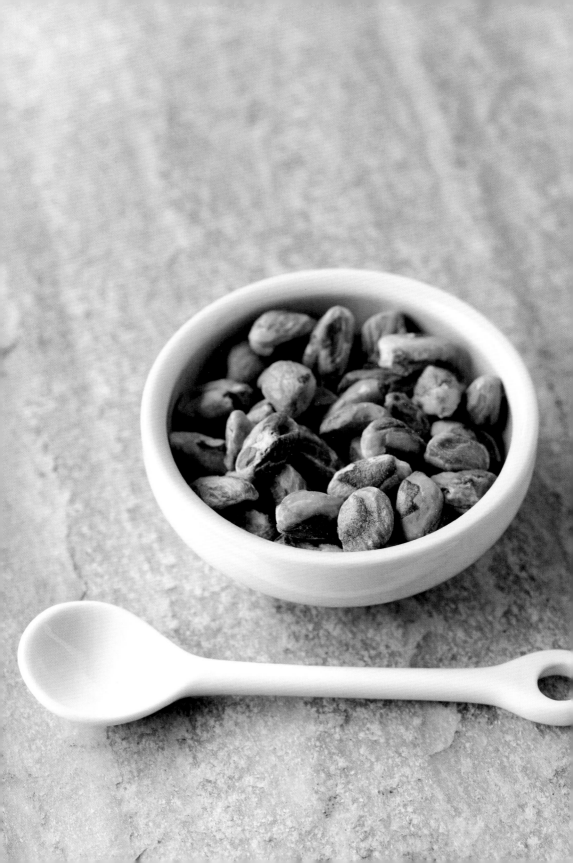

PISTACHIO NUT

THE HEART'S BEST FRIEND.

■ **ACTIVE INGREDIENTS**

The pistachio nut contains an appreciable amount of protein, unsaturated fatty acids and phytosterols recognized for their beneficial effects on blood lipids.

■ **PROPERTIES**

Several epidemiological and clinical studies link regular consumption of tree nuts, including pistachios, to various health benefits, mainly on the cardiovascular system, thanks to the presence of unsaturated fatty acids and phytosterols. Pistachios also contain vitamins and resveratrol, a powerful antioxidant also beneficial for the prevention of cardiovascular disease and to fight against ageing.

■ **USE**

As accompaniment to salads, meats, and desserts.

■ **PRECAUTIONS**

Avoid if allergic to peanuts.

■ **FOR THE RECORD ...**

According to legend, the Queen of Sheba decreed that pistachios were food exclusively reserved for royalty and went to prevent the people to grow them for their personal use.

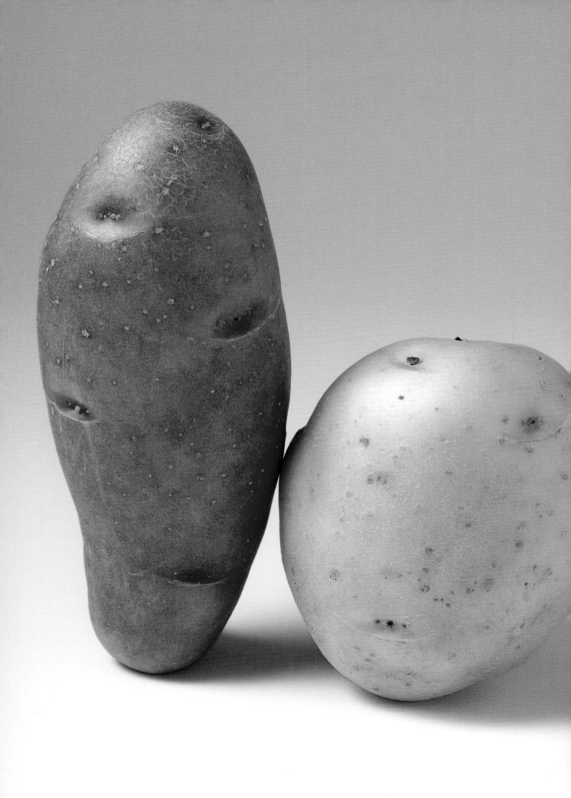

POTATO

A COMPLETE FOOD.

◼ ACTIVE INGREDIENTS

The potato is a complete food. It is rich in vitamins of groups B and C, flavonoids (in an amount more important in purple potatoes), minerals and trace elements like potassium, magnesium, iron, zinc, copper, and fiber.

◼ PROPERTIES

The potato cells protect against attacks from free radicals.
Easily digestible, it is suitable for all ages.
It is known to be part of the foods that can fight cancer.
It helps lower the «bad» cholesterol, and promotes digestion.

◼ USE

La Ratte, russet, Yukon gold… potatoes are available all year depending on the variety. Choose them with a skin that is smooth, without black or green spots. Make sure they do not contain germs. They will keep several days protected from light and heat.

No contraindication.

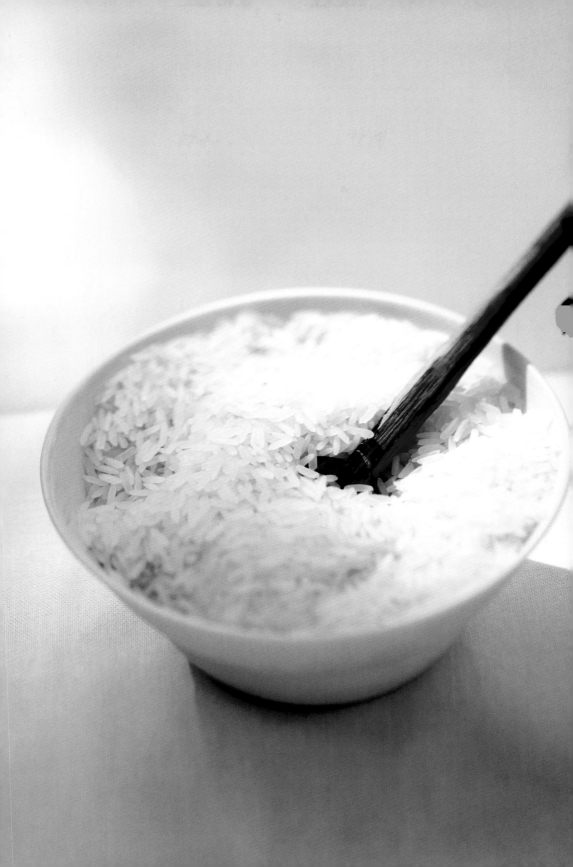

RICE

A SOURCE OF ENERGY.

■ ACTIVE INGREDIENTS

Brown rice is richer, has not undergone any process of refining which is responsible for the loss of many nutrients. It is a source of magnesium, manganese, selenium, fiber, B vitamins, E. All varieties of rice are devoid of gluten.

■ PROPERTIES

Brown rice provides energy during the day.
It promotes digestion and fights constipation.
It would have the power to decrease the «bad» cholesterol, and is believed to fight cancer.
White rice and the water in which it was cooked are believed to stop diarrhea.
Rice is suitable for people with celiac disease.

■ USE

Different kinds of rice are commercially available, including basmati, brown rice, Arborio, red rice, and wild rice ...
Rice will keep for several months in a dry place in a container tightly closed, away from light.
There are many foods on the market derived from Rice: a rice drink (commonly called rice «milk»), patties, puffed rice, rice flour (alternative to wheat in cases of intolerance to gluten), rice noodles, rice oil.

No contraindication.

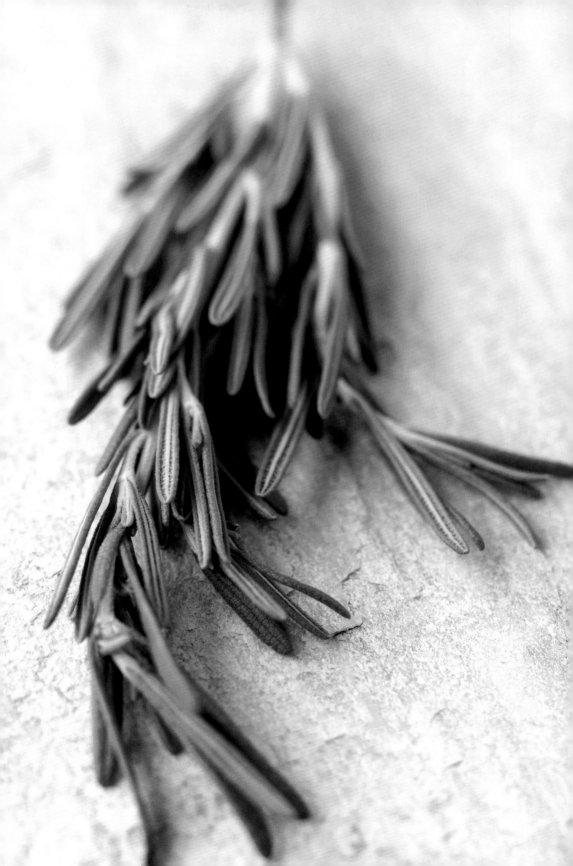

ROSEMARY

GOOD FOR THE LIVER.

■ **ACTIVE INGREDIENTS**

It is full of flavonoids.

■ **PROPERTIES**

Rosemary is an outstanding ally for those who suffer from liver problems and gastro-intestinal problems. It acts at the level of the gallbladder, increasing the secretion of bile and facilitating its discharge into the intestine. It is recommended for rheumatism, fatigue, dizziness and nervous disorders of the general kind. Rosemary is also present in almost all stress-relieving teas: for a better sleep and for being in a good mood after waking up well etc…

■ **USE**

In herb form to accompany meat and fish, and as an infusion (2 g of dried rosemary per 150 ml of water). Rosemary exists as liquid extract.

No contraindication.

■ **FOR THE RECORD …**

The Greeks used it to enhance memory and stimulate the intellect. A fact noted by two preliminary studies performed on subjects exposed to the essential oil in rosemary.

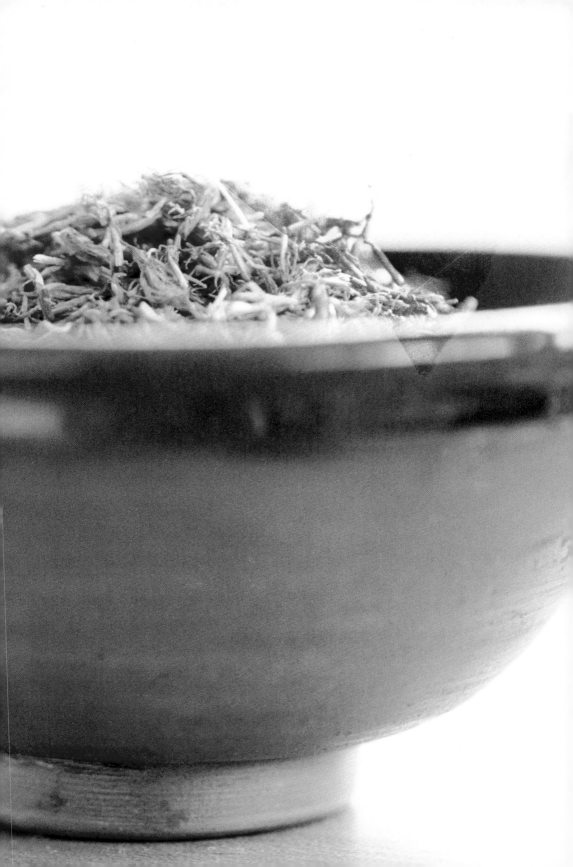

SAFFRON

THE YELLOW GOLD.

ACTIVE INGREDIENTS

Saffron contains safranal, a volatile oil responsible for its aroma, and contains carotenoids of which the crocin gives it its yellow-orange color.

PROPERTIES

Saffron is one of the plants richest in riboflavin, or vitamin B, a water-soluble vitamin necessary for the proper functioning of the nervous system. Safranal has many stimulant virtues that make it a good antidepressant. Along with crocin, which gives a yellow-gold tone to food, another carotenoid picrocrocin, plays a protective role against free radicals.
Saffron is known to aid digestion.

USE

It is in the form of powder or fibers and enters the composition of many culinary specialties.

No contraindication.

FOR THE RECORD ...

Powdered saffron is obtained by harvesting and drying the stamens of Crocus sativus which were handpicked. It takes about 200,000 stigmas to produce one kilogram of the precious purple toned gold and 5 kg of fresh stamens to obtain 1kg of dried saffron.

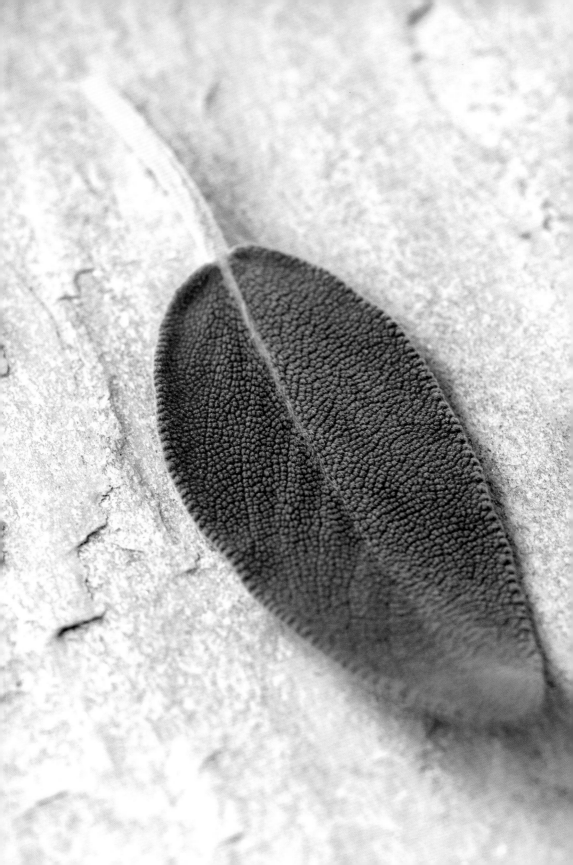

SAGE

ROYALLY TASTY WITH HONEY.

ACTIVE INGREDIENTS

Sage contains an essential oil rich in estrogen, in flavonoids and tannins.

PROPERTIES

Sage exerts a detoxifying effect on the liver and kidneys.
It is anti-diarrheal agent and facilitates menstruation. During premenopause, it regulates the cycles and reduces hot flashes. It also has the property of triggering perspiration, which is why we recommend it during influenza and fevers. A daily infusion of sage, sweetened with honey, would greatly relieve asthma sufferers.

USE

Can be used as a seasoning in stews, sauces and on deli meats.
As an infusion: 30 g of dried sage to one liter of water. Infuse a quarter of an hour.

No contraindication.

FOR THE RECORD ...

Sage was "salvia salvatrix" in latin, the plant that saves and heals. Its powers are immortalized in the aphorism of the famous School of Salerno: "Cur moriatur homo, cui salvia in Crescit Horto? («Why does a man die when sage grows inhis garden? «)
Moreover, the Latin name for sage, "salvia" means «health».

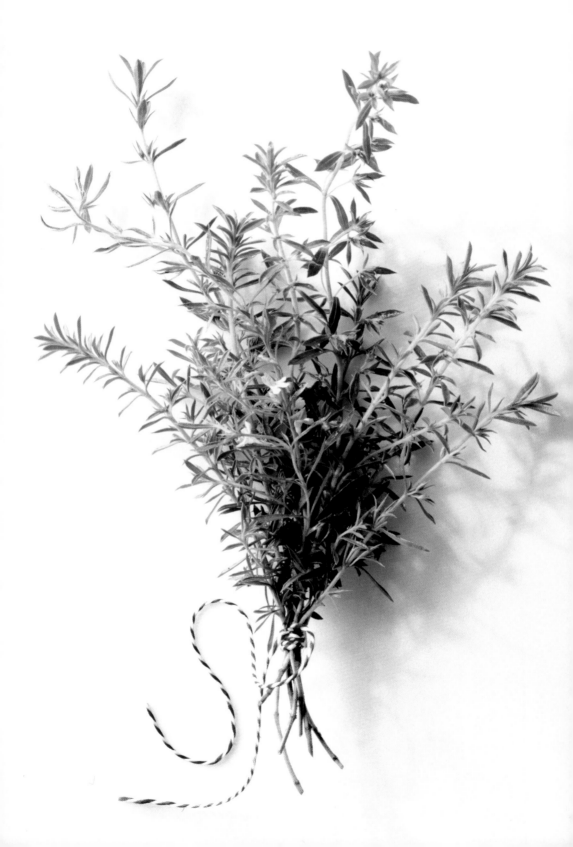

SAVORY

THE DIGESTION HERB.

■ ACTIVE INGREDIENTS

Unlike fine herbs, savory is a source of antioxidants and nutrients (iron, manganese, calcium, magnesium and vitamin B6).

■ PROPERTIES

Antioxidants are an ally in the prevention of cardiovascular diseases and diseases related to ageing.
Extracts and the essential oil in savory have been seen to have antifungal effects, antibacterial, anti-inflammatory, analgesic, antispasmodic and anti-diarrheal effects.

■ USE

As a seasoning for food use. Drops, by oral ingestion or as an essential oil.

■ PRECAUTIONS

Ask a doctor in case of blood-thinning treatment.
Do not use the pure essential oil.

■ FOR THE RECORD ...

The leaves are used since ancient times, to add flavor to grilled meats but also to help digestion and avoid bloating and gas. The Romans believed it to be an aphrodisiac, which earned it the name "satyr grass".

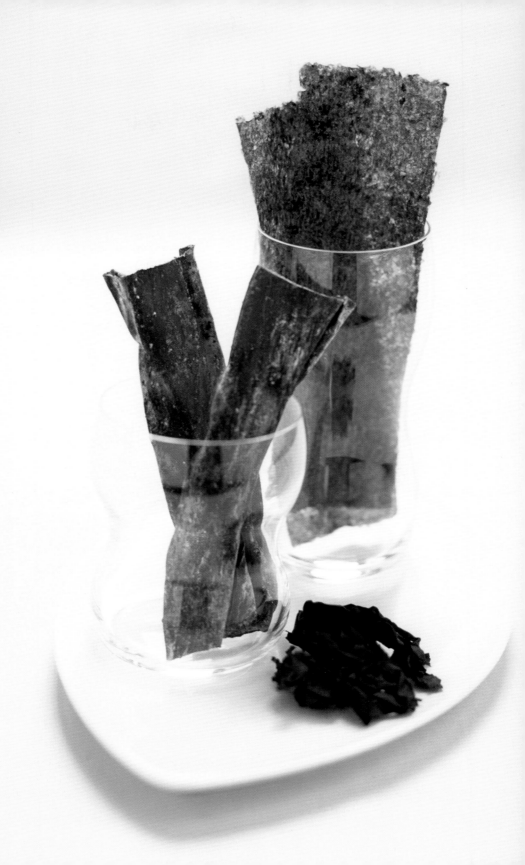

SEAWEED

TOXIN TRAPS.

■ ACTIVE INGREDIENT

Each type of seaweed has specific characteristics but they are all a great source of nutrients.

They are rich in minerals and trace elements (approximately 25% of their weight), in calcium (iziki and wakame), in magnesium (wakame, nori, sea lettuce, dulse), in iron (sea lettuce, dulse, iziki), in phosphorus (nori) and many others (iodine, potassium, sulfur, chrome, zinc, cobalt, sodium, manganese…).

They also contain many vitamins : of the B, C and A groups.

The protein content varies according to seaweed quality but it is estimated at 20% of the total weight.

■ PROPERTIES

Thanks to the presence of a component, algin, they are toxins traps, that is to say that they facilitate the elimination of wastes in our body.

They facilitate digestion, thanks to the fiber they contain.

They stimulate our body's natural defenses and have mineralizing powers thanks to the large amount of minerals and trace elements in them.

■ USE

You find seaweed in natural food stores and natural products stores. They can be fresh, preserved in a thin layer of salt, or dried whole leaf, chopped or as flakes. When they are fresh, they keep only a few days in the refrigerator. If dried, they keep well in a dry place, away from light. They can also be frozen.

■ PRECAUTIONS

Seaweed should be eaten in small quantities, bur regularly.

Because of the presence of iodine, persons suffering from thyroid problems should seek advice from their doctor before making significant use of it.

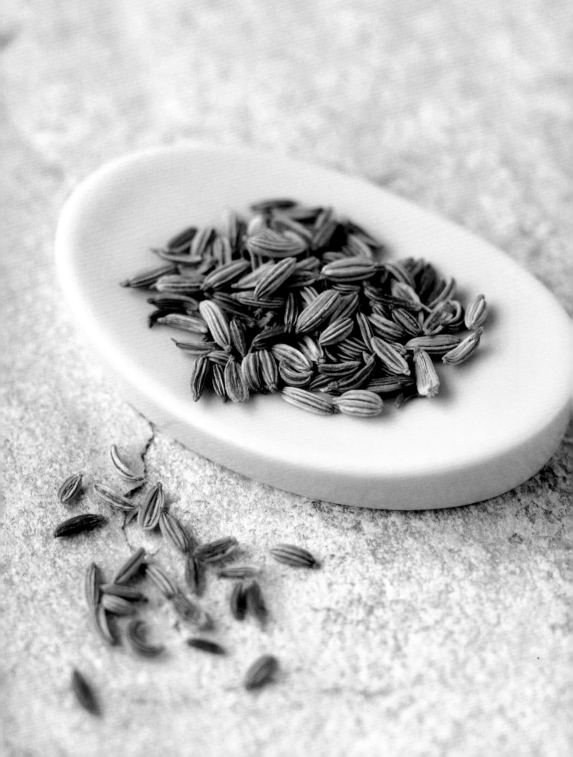

SESAME

VALUABLE LITTLE SEEDS.

ACTIVE INGREDIENTS

The sesame seed is a concentrate of protein, minerals and valuable trace elements. Lecithin, a phosphorus compound, is of great value to the nervous system, to the endocrine glands and to sexual function.

PROPERTIES

It is primarily a powerful re-mineralizing agent. The presence of sesamol also gives it antioxidant and digestive properties.

The sesame seed is one of the foods that contain a high concentration of phytosterols, which are beneficial for cardiovascular health, because they reduce LDL («bad» cholesterol). Studies are underway for determining what could be its use in geriatrics and on its action on the central nervous system as an anxiolytic and an anti-stress agent.

USE

As seasoning in seed form or in oil form.

PRECAUTIONS

Avoid if allergic.

FOR THE RECORD ...

In India, sesame seeds are a symbol of immortality.

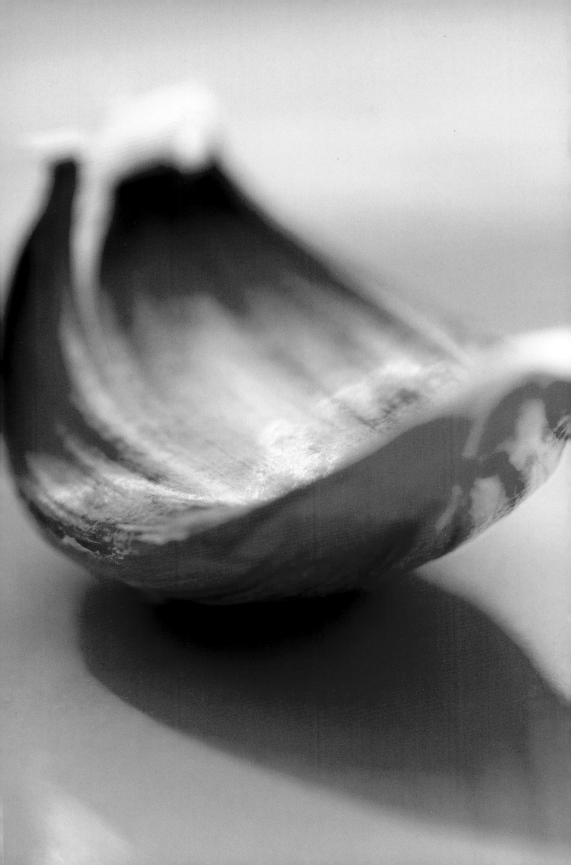

SHALLOT

ANTIOXIDANTS IN THE BULB.

ACTIVE INGREDIENTS

The strong antioxidant activity in shallots is attributed to the flavonoids and beta-carotene they contain.
They are also a very good source of vitamins and trace elements.

PROPERTIES

Antioxidants protect the body against free radicals, the molecules involved in cardiovascular diseases, certain cancers and other diseases related to ageing.
Shallots also contain sulfur compounds that would mainly have a protective effect in digestive tract cancers. The shallot is also known for its antimicrobial and antifungal effects.

USE

The bulbs are used raw or cooked, or as solids.

No contraindication.

FOR THE RECORD ...

There are onions and shallots: until 1990, only shallots, considered noble and traditional, were allowed to be marketed under the name shallots. It is only since then that the seeds can legitimately bear this name.

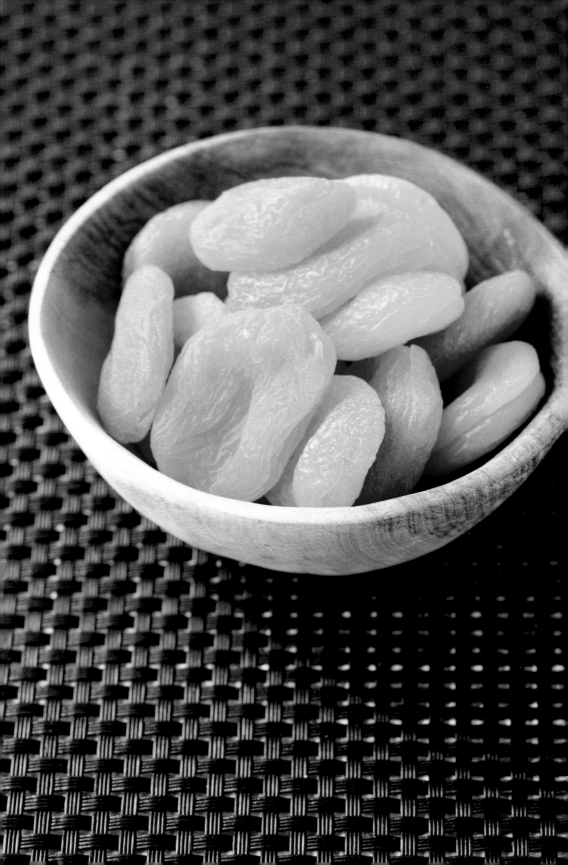

SOFT DRIED FRUITS

A GREAT SOURCE OF ENERGY.

■ ACTIVE INGREDIENTS

A freshly picked fruit contains about 80% water.
Once dried, it becomes a treasure trove of minerals and valuable trace elements, including phosphorus, calcium, iron and potassium in large quantity, as well as vitamins, sugars and fibers.
With regard to vitamins, only vitamin C (too fragile) disappears during the drying process, except in bananas that are dried, while there remains vitamins A and B in considerable quantities,

■ PROPERTIES

Regular use of soft dried fruits reduces the consumption of refined sugar.
They are a source of immediate energy, as they contain sucrose, fructose or glucose, which are useful when you are tired.
They promote bowel movements.

■ USE

Dried fruits keep well in a jar tightly closed away from heat and light.
It is wiser to buy organic fruits, to be sure the drying process used is natural and not chemical, in order for the fruits to keep all their nutritional value.

■ PRECAUTIONS

Because they contain quite a few calories, they are to be eaten in moderate quantities.

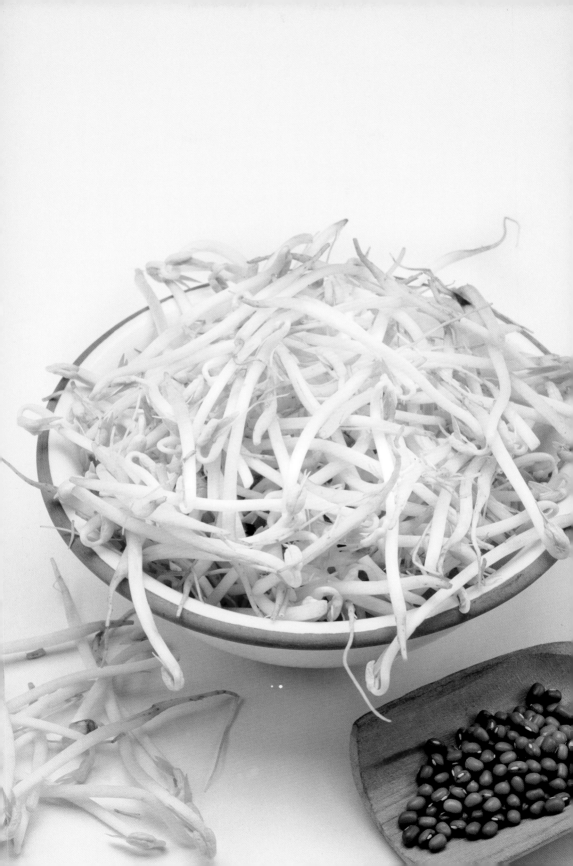

SOYBEAN

A LEGUME FULL OF VIRTUES!

■ ACTIVE INGREDIENTS

Rich in vegetable protein (about 37% of its weight), soybean contains fiber, unsaturated fatty acids, vitamins of the B group, minerals and trace elements like calcium, magnesium, iron, manganese, zinc, copper, selenium and phosphorus. Soy contains isoflavones that have a role similar to estrogen. It is therefore believed that soy contains phytoestrogens. It is also a source of lecithin, found in brain cells.

■ PROPERTIES

Soybeans may reduce the risk of cardiovascular disease.
Soy reduces the levels of «bad» cholesterol.
It is effective against the inconveniences of the menopause. It is a food that can help fight cancer, particularly breast cancer. It has a positive effect on blood pressure. With the amount of fiber, it promotes intestinal transit and prevents constipation. It prevents mental fatigue.
It stimulates the immune system.

■ USE

Soy comes in a multitude of products: seeds, shoots, «milk», flour, cooking cream, tofu, pasta, ice cream ...

■ PRECAUTIONS

Some subjects are allergic to soy.
Beware: soy is going through important changes on the genetic level. This is one of the plants most involved in the controversy on GMOs. Make sure it is from an organic source or marked «GMO free».

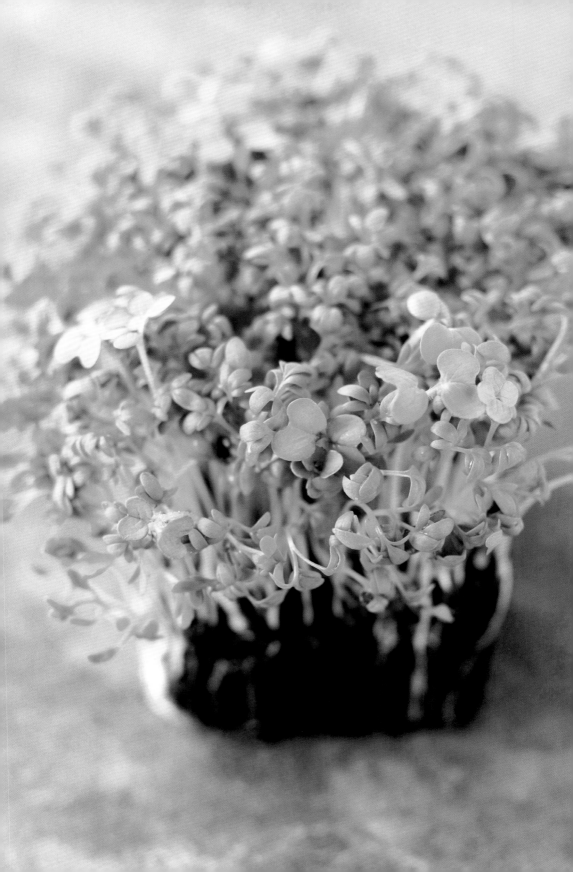

SPROUTS

ACTIVE INGREDIENTS

During germination, the number of vitamins (A, B, C, E) and minerals (calcium, iron, magnesium, potassium, zinc, phosphorus...) contained in each seed increases dramatically.

For example, vitamins increase from 50 to 100%. Protein and other nutrients are reduced to be better assimilated by the body. Chlorophyll, which is to say, the green pigment found in plants, is growing considerably.

PROPERTIES

Sprouts are mineralizing.

Energy-boosting, they give a boost when you are tired and suffer from a general sense of apathy.

They purify the body of accumulated toxins, promote better digestion and fight stomach acid.

They are allowed when dieting.

They are suitable for all ages, particularly for the elderly, for children, the convalescing and pregnant women.

USE

Buy sprouts ready in specialized health food stores or where they are guaranteed pesticide free and free of other chemicals.

You can easily germinate seeds at home using a plastic or terra cotta propagator. To germinate, they need darkness, moisture, air and a warm place. Let the seeds soak in water overnight. Rinse the next day. When still wet, let the seeds remain another day in the dark. Repeat for 3 to 5 days.

The germination time is variable depending on the seed used.

Gradually, the shoots begin to appear, white at first, then green with a significantly higher concentration chlorophyll.

No contraindication.

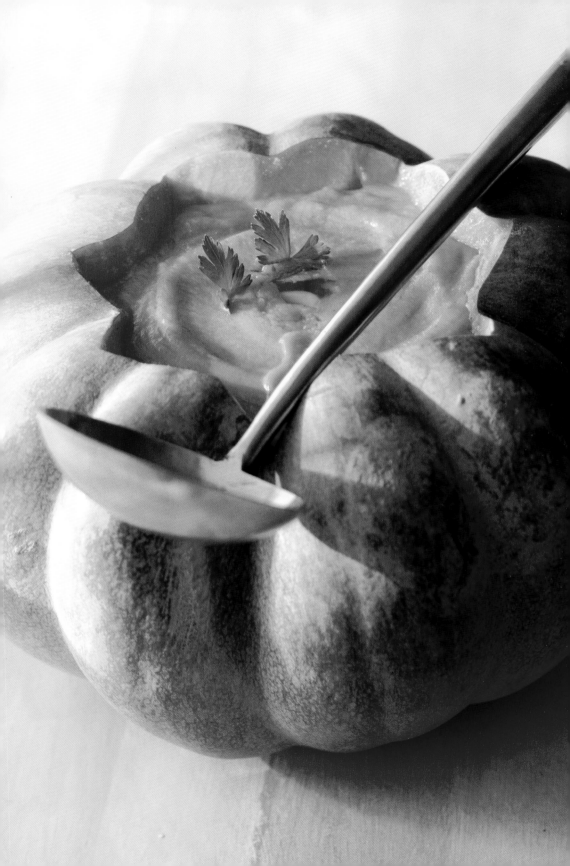

SQUASH

FIGHTS CELLULAR AGEING.

ACTIVE INGREDIENTS

Rich in provitamin A, squash contains vitamins B and C, fiber, minerals and trace elements (iron, manganese, copper) and other antioxidants.

PROPERTIES

Squash helps prevent cardiovascular diseases.
It contributes to the maintenance of healthy skin.
It is suitable for diets.
Squash seeds are used to combat worms.
Seeds and seed oil help prevent prostate disorders.

USE

Enjoy it every month as squash comes in different varieties of the same family, the Cucurbitaceous: the butternut squash, the spaghetti squash, the lettuce squash, and the buttercup.
Whole, they will keep several weeks at room temperature (up to about three months) or longer if they are stored in a cellar. If they are cut, they must be kept in the crisper of the refrigerator. Once cooked squash can be frozen.

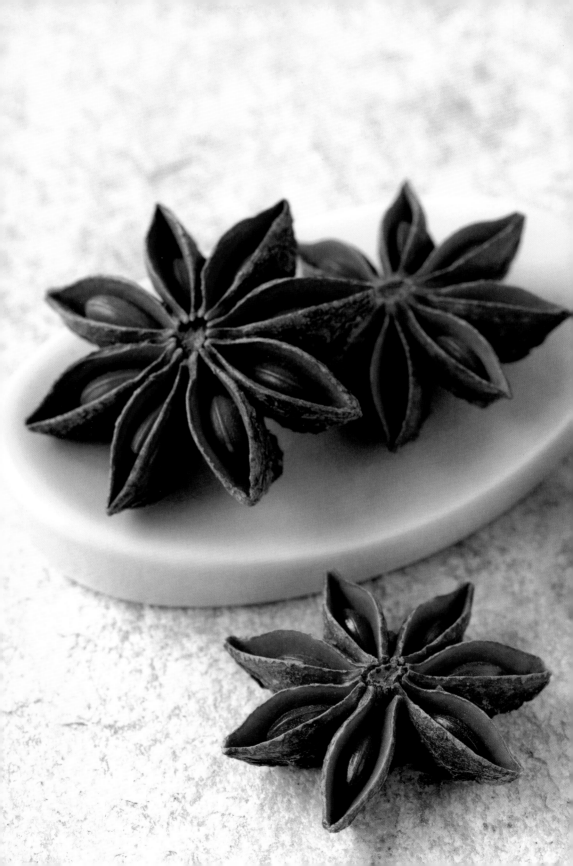

STAR ANISE

A GOOD INTESTINAL ANTISEPTIC.

■ ACTIVE INGREDIENTS

The essential oil of the badianier tree contains anethole (who gives it its flavor) and tannins.

■ PROPERTIES

In Europe, the fruit of the badianier tree is mainly used in the manufacture of Pastis, the French anise-based alcoholic drink. It has stomach-relieving properties, as well as carminative and antispasmodic properties. It is a good intestinal antiseptic.

■ USE

Some seeds are sufficient to flavor a dish. Widely used in Chinese cuisine, star anise is a component of the «five flavors», with Szechuan pepper, fennel, cloves and cinnamon. As an infusion it eliminates bloating, reduces gas (10 to 15 minutes after each meal).
In capsule form (dry): 300 mg with a glass of water after each meal.

No contraindication.

■ FOR THE RECORD ...

Chinese star anise is used in the manufacture of shikimic acid, which, after several transformations, becomes Oseltamivir phosphate, the active molecule of Tamiflu, a flu vaccine.

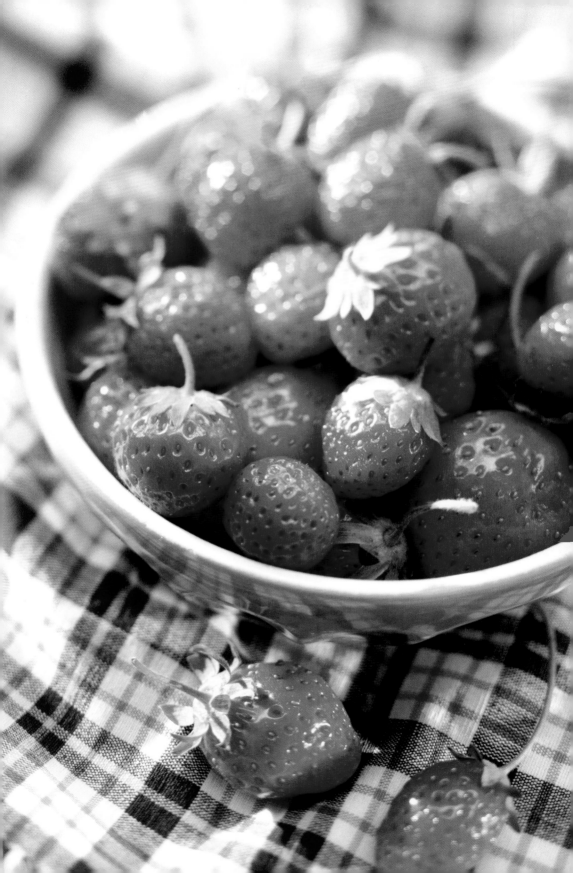

STRAWBERRY

A FRIEND TO THE SKIN.

ACTIVE INGREDIENTS

Strawberry is rich in vitamins, the most interesting being vitamin C. It also contains fiber, vitamin B, provitamin A, minerals and trace elements, such as potassium, calcium, magnesium, iron, fluorine, and cobalt.

PROPERTIES

The strawberry is a friend of the skin.
It helps fight viral and bacterial infections.
It protects blood vessel walls.
It is a good depurative and has diuretic qualities.
It stimulates the immune system.

USE

Buy strawberries ripe, firm, bright red with bright green stalks. They must be eaten quickly because they will keep only 2 days in the crisper.
Large-sized Strawberries are often sipped with water and do not have much taste.

PRECAUTIONS

Strawberries frequently cause allergies in some people who are sensitive to its chemical make-up.

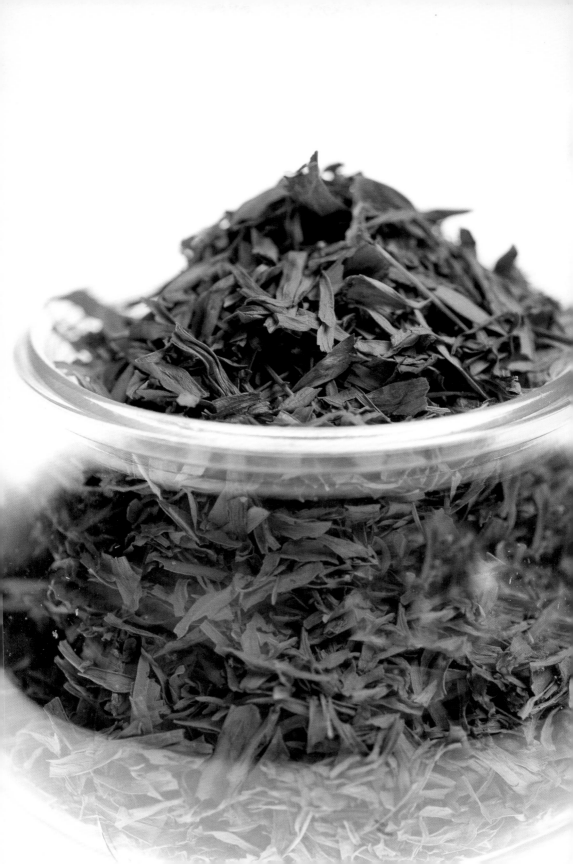

TARRAGON

WITH ANXIOLYTIC EFFECT.

■ **ACTIVE INGREDIENTS**

Besides antioxidants, researchers found in extracts of tarragon, the presence of benzodiazepines which have act on the central nervous system.

■ **PROPERTIES**

Some antioxidants such as flavonoids, contained in tarragon may act as anti-allergenic agents. The presence of benzodiazepines also suggests that tarragon may possess anxiolytic effects, but in the absence of scientific evidence, we cannot imagine replacing synthetic benzodiazepine with tarragon.

■ **USE**

As an accompaniment, it is used fresh or dried.

■ **PRECAUTIONS**

The presence of vitamin K requires the opinion of a physician or pharmacist if blood-thinning treatment is taken.

■ **FOR THE RECORD ...**

Its name which means dragon, or dragon-grass, is very likely given this herb because of the shape of its roots similar to a snake. Serendipity: the Greeks and Romans used it for treating snakebites.

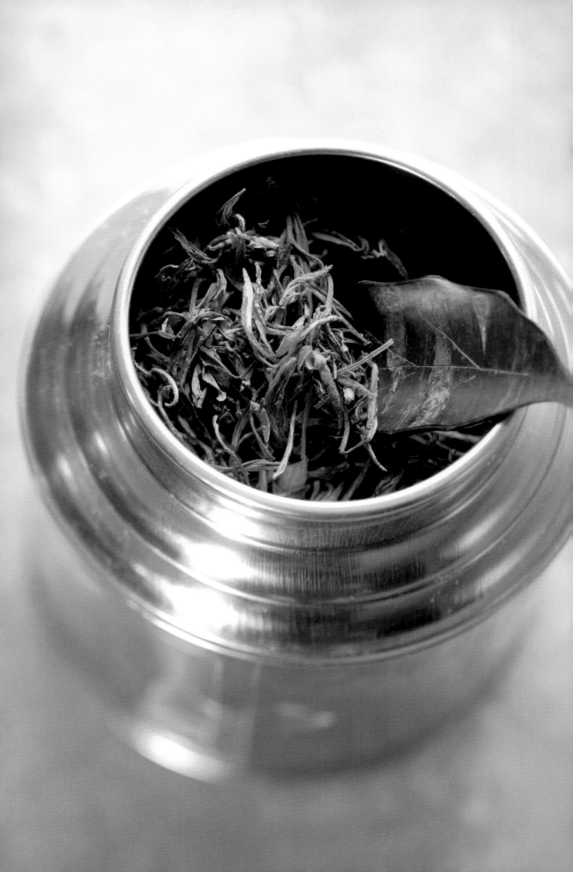

TEA

ALL YOU CAN DRINK!

■ ACTIVE INGREDIENTS

It contains caffeine, polyphenols, proteins and minerals.

■ PROPERTIES

Tea helps fight against free radicals responsible for ageing and nearly all age-related diseases (cardiovascular, cancer, cataracts, arthritis, Parkinson's and Alzheimer's). It has an anti-inflammatory effect, is an attention booster, stimulates concentration, it promotes the burning of fat in adipose tissue.
We can drink as much tea as we want because it has no calories.

■ USE

Tea is almost a universal drink which can be drunk with or in between meals. Let steep for at least 5 minutes. It can accompany any recipe.

■ PRECAUTIONS

Avoid drinking tea if you are anemic.

■ FOR THE RECORD ....

There are lots of legends around tea: the best known one is from 2374 BC. The Chinese monarch, Chen-nung, would put water to boil to drink in the shade of a bush.
Under the effect of a light wind, some dry leaves fell into his hot water. Tasting the water, he was surprised by the flavor and the aroma it had acquired.

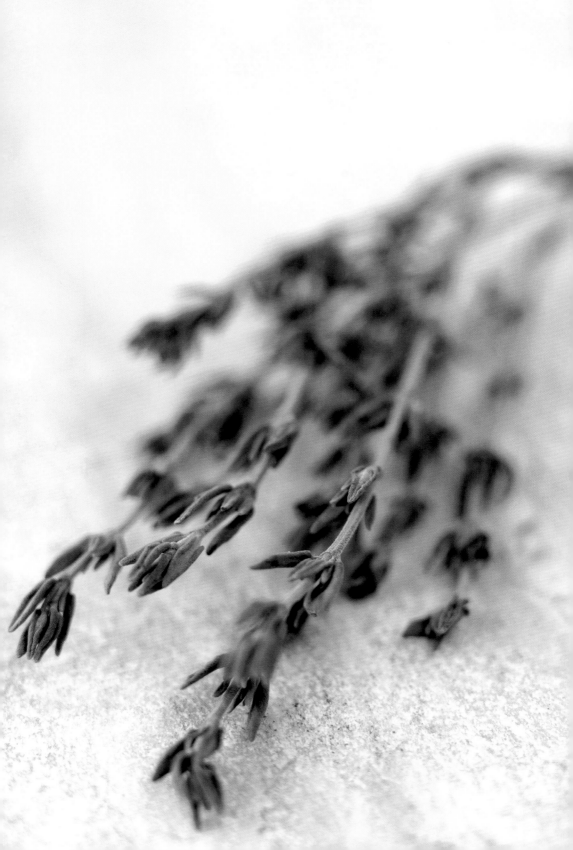

THYME

A MUST OF PROVENCAL CUISINE.

■ ACTIVE INGREDIENTS

Thyme contains an essential oil containing thymol, flavonoids and tannins.

■ PROPERTIES

Thyme is one of the plants most recommended by the European Commission against cough and inflammation of the upper respiratory tract. It is a good disinfectant and an antiseptic. The WHO mentions it in the treatment of dyspepsia and other gastro-intestinal disorders. Research on animals have allowed us to observe its antioxidant antiplatelet and relaxing as well as antifungal properties.

■ USE

Fresh or dried for flavoring dishes.
As an infusion for cough: 10 g of dried thyme per liter of water, let steep 5 minutes. Drink 250 to 500 ml per day.
Exists in the form of essential oil.

■ PRECAUTIONS

Consider the presence of vitamin K. It is responsible for Allergies to thyme.

■ FOR THE RECORD ...

The Romans filled their beds with it to enjoy a better sleep. The custom is that a sprig of thyme slipped under the pillow helps us sleep better still persists.

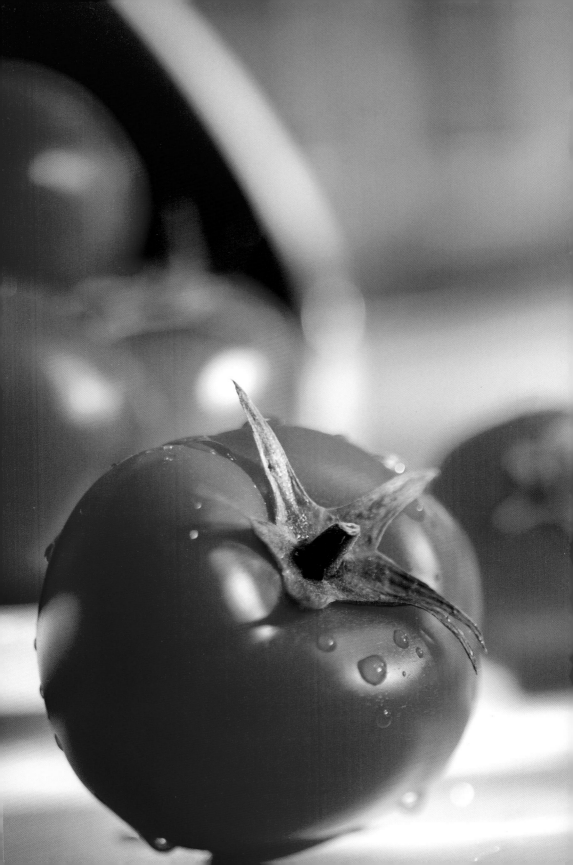

TOMATO

FIGHTS THE AGEING OF CELLS.

ACTIVE INGREDIENTS

Tomatoes contain lycopenes, powerful antioxidants that are allies in the prevention of prostate disorders. They also contain fiber, other antioxidants, vitamins C and E, beta-carotene, minerals and trace elements, as potassium, magnesium, and calcium.

PROPERTIES

The tomato plants are believed to have the ability to help fight cancer formation.
It prevents disease and cardiovascular disease and blood clots.
It helps fight the «bad» cholesterol.
It is beneficial to the prostate.
It stimulates the digestive secretions.

USE

Choose ripe but firm tomatoes, uniform in color and ones that smell good. They will keep at room temperature for a few days. In the refrigerator, they have a longer shelf life, but they lose some of their flavor.
Tomatoes can also be bought canned - whole, crushed, as coulis, as concentrate - or dried.

PRECAUTIONS

It can cause allergies or be badly tolerated. Its seeds may cause irritation.

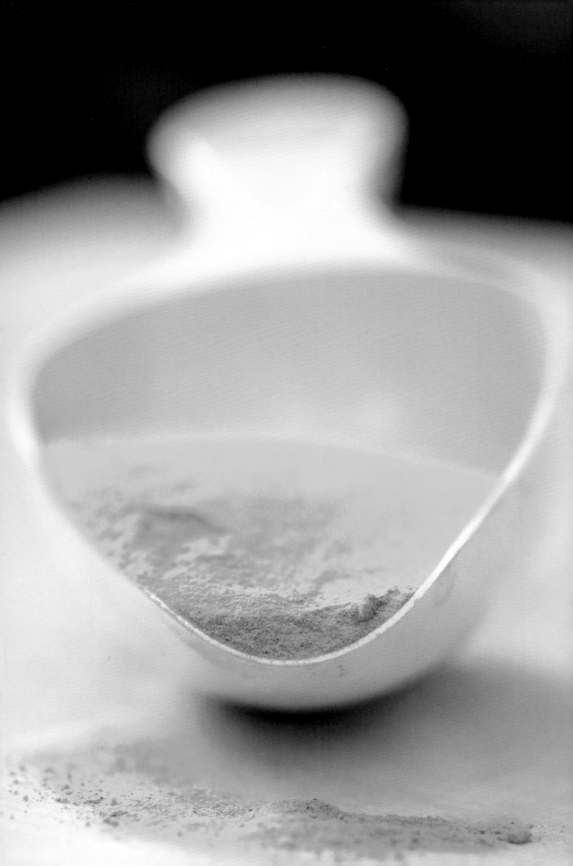

TURMERIC

ACTIVE INGREDIENTS

The plant is rich in phenolic pigments, the curcuminoids (Represented by 90% curcumin) which are antioxidants very powerful.

PROPERTIES

The World Health Organization (WHO) acknowledges the efficiency of turmeric in the treatment of some digestive disorders, as stomach upset, loss of appetite or the sensation of being stuffed and or bloated.

The presence of curcumin could explain a number of therapeutic properties, including its anti-inflammatory (relief of rheumatism and arthritis pain, and the treatment of skin disorders inflammatory ophthalmological pain). The antioxidant effect of curcumin also allows us to see its protective effect against oxidative stress-related illnesses, such as cardiovascular disease and Alzheimer's disease. Turmeric is finally believed to play a protective role against some cancers: for example, epidemiological data indicate that the occurrence of colon cancer is much lower in countries where turmeric is heavily consumed.

USE

It comes in powder form. This is the basic ingredient for the composition of curry. Available in capsules: take three to six per day.

PRECAUTIONS

Ask a Doctor in case of gastric ulcer or gallstones before taking turmeric capsules. In cases of high consumption, turmeric may have an blood-thinning effect.

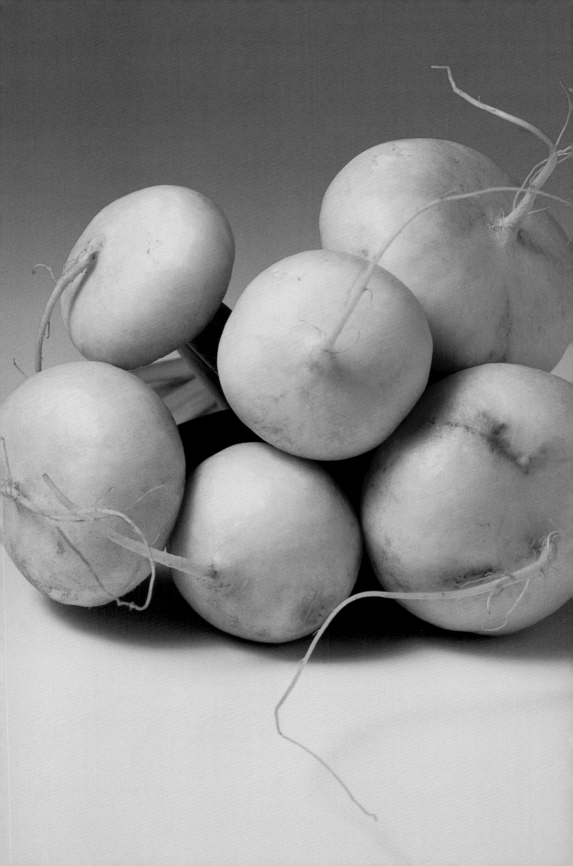

TURNIP

ACTIVE INGREDIENTS

There are lots of antioxidants, vitamin B, C, fiber, minerals and trace elements like iron, manganese, phosphorus, magnesium, potassium, copper, and sulfur in the turnip.

PROPERTIES

Would be part of the vegetables that help fight cancer.
It helps in cough and phlegm.
It helps fight the proliferation of free radicals in part responsible of aging.
This is a good diuretic.

USE

Turnips are sold in bunches at markets in the spring.
The turnip (spring or fall turnip) should have a smooth glossy skin and should not be too light. It keeps about twelve days in the crisper.

PRECAUTIONS

Turnips can cause bloating in stomachs that are sensitive.

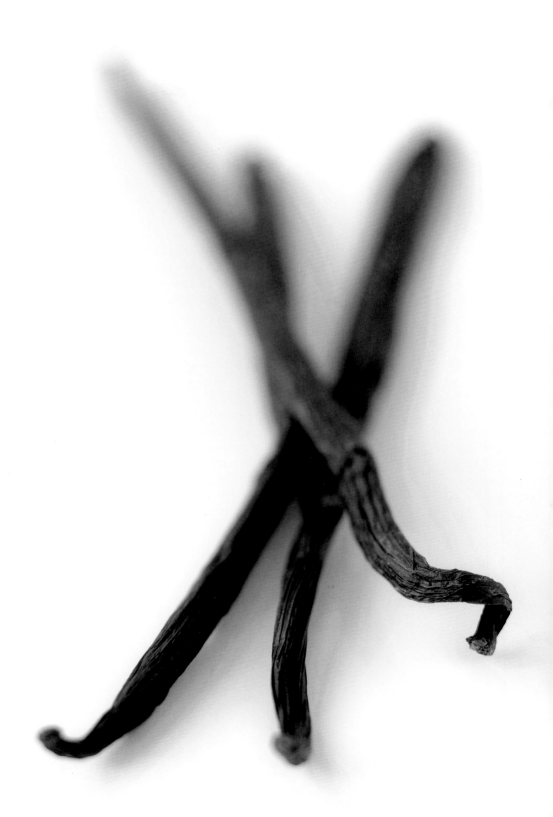

VANILLA

REPUTED TO BE AN APHRODISIAC.

■ ACTIVE INGREDIENTS

Vanillin gives the flavor and properties of various vanillas.

■ PROPERTIES

Vanilla is world renowned for its aphrodisiac properties. It is effective in the fight against stress and "the blues". It also has antiseptic properties.
Unusual fact: it could have a weight loss effect: patches with vanilla, placed on the back of the hand, are currently at the testing stage.

■ USE

Pods, liquid extract or powdered for flavoring dishes. Enters into the composition of many herbal teas.

No contraindication.

■ FOR THE RECORD ...

In some parts of South America, men macerate some vanilla beans in white alcohol for nearly a month ... and claim that with 15 drops of this mixture every day, they are... exceptionally fit.

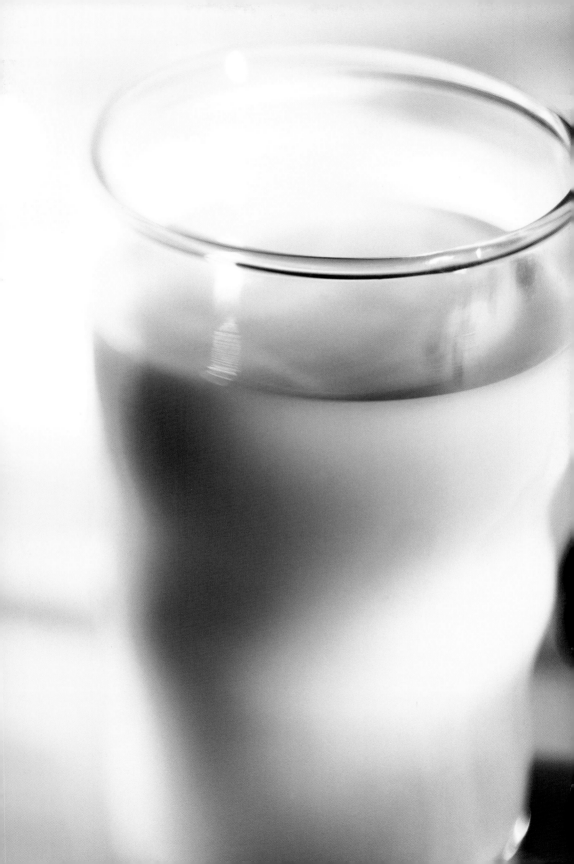

VEGETABLE «MILKS»

ACTIVE INGREDIENTS

It contains minerals such as calcium, magnesium, vitamins, fiber, carbohydrates and some protein in larger or smaller quantity depending on the variety of milk.

PROPERTIES

Beverages made from cereals are lactose and cholesterol-free some are also gluten-free (such as those that are rice or quinoa-based).
Soy beverages, chestnut and fruit seed oils (hazelnut and almond) contain no cholesterol or lactose or gluten.

USE

"Tetrapacked" like cow's milk or as single servings, vegetable «milks» are purchased ready for use in health food stores, as well as in most supermarkets. These drinks are sold plain or flavored (i.e. vanilla and chocolate).
Some of them chestnut or almond milks can be purchased in powder form or as paste which dissolve in water to obtain the desired beverage.
Choose beverages labeled «organic farming».
That guarantees the absence of GMOs and chemicals in the culture and manufacturing processes.

PRECAUTIONS

From a nutritional standpoint, vegetable milks should not replace milk by a cow because they contain far fewer proteins for example.

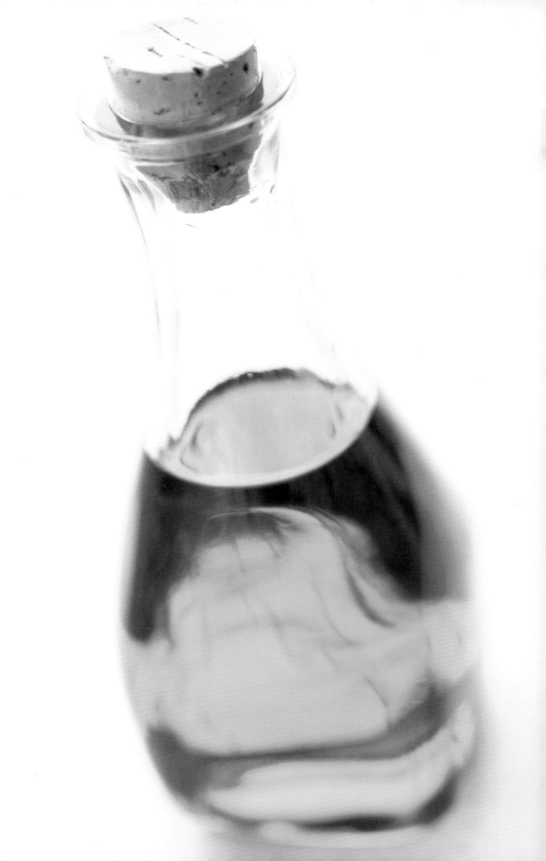

VEGETABLE OILS

ESSENTIAL TO THE BODY.

ACTIVE INGREDIENTS

Vegetable oils contain thousands of fatty acids unsaturated omega-3 (especially walnut oil, rapeseed oil and hemp oil) and omega-6, polyphenols (especially olive oil)
Vitaamin A and E (especially sunflower oil).

PROPERTIES

Vegetable oils protect the cardiovascular system and prevent unrest.
They help reduce levels of «bad» cholesterol.
They have antioxidant and fight the ageing of cells.
They promote bowel movements.
They feed the cells of the nervous system and brain.

USE

Choose cold-pressed vegetable oils!
Avoid refined oils.
Keep oils away from light, if possible in opaque glass containers and away from humidity. Oils deteriorate when they are subject to oxidation.

PRECAUTIONS

To retain all their properties, vegetable oils must be eaten raw.

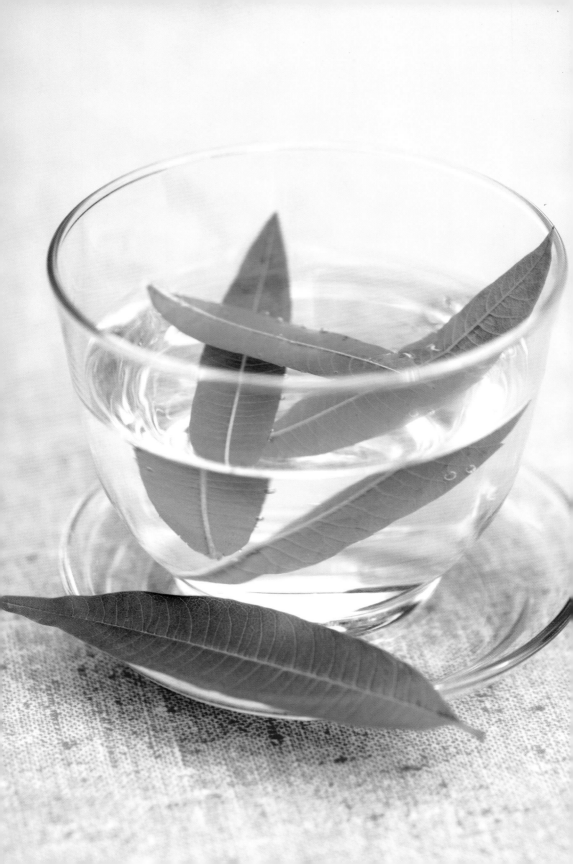

VERBENA

SACRED HERB BY THE ROMANS.

■ **ACTIVE INGREDIENTS**

The most important is the verbenalin. There are also tannins, mucilage, saponin and quinones.

■ **PROPERTIES**

The plant has neuralgic properties thanks to the verbenalin and to its other compounds it owes its fever-reducing and anti inflammatory properties.
It is a tonic, an antispasmodic (useful against nervousness, coughs, insomnia, and anxiety).

■ **USE**

In conventional brewing: two to three cups per day for its sedative properties. It is also an excellent remedy for diseases of the eye.
Boil the leaves in vinegar, two handfuls of verbena for a liter of vinegar: put a cloth soaked with it and apply as a compress on the your sides, kidney or forehead for headaches.
For gargling because of an inflammation of the mouth, or as compresses, it will be used to soothe wounds, cuts and lymph rashes and bruises.

No contraindication.

■ **FOR THE RECORD ...**

In ancient Gaul, the druid gave verbena ownership of the power to cure all diseases, to destroy evil, and to inspire gaiety.

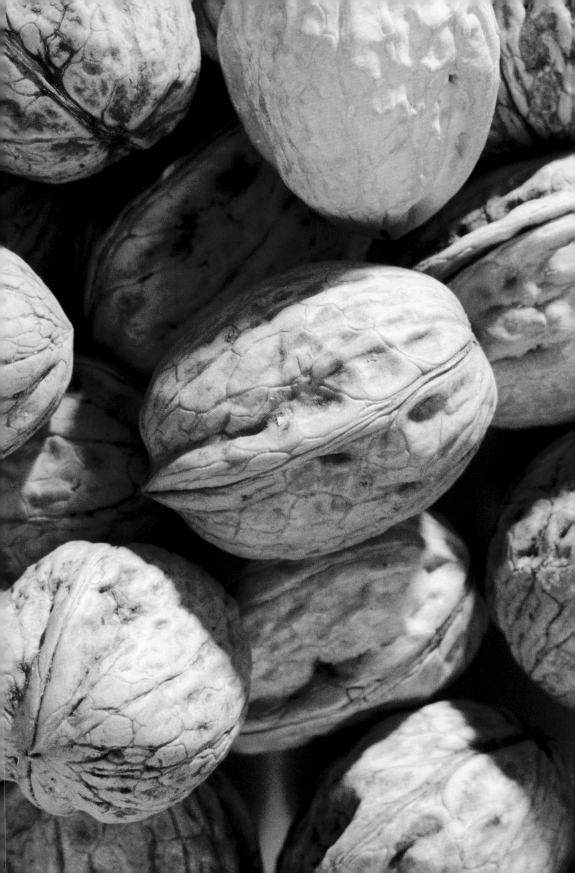

WALNUT

A GOOD SOURCE OF OMEGA-3.

■ ACTIVE INGREDIENTS

Particularly rich in polyunsaturated fatty acids, the walnut is a food that contains plenty of omega-3. It contains many antioxidant, melatonin, fibers, vegetable proteins, minerals and trace elements such as manganese, phosphorus, magnesium, iron, vitamins B and E.

■ PROPERTIES

It is beneficial to cardiovascular health because it is believed to have a protective action against the problems related to blood flow.
It reduces levels of «bad» cholesterol.
Its high fiber content helps digestion.
It promotes the proper functioning of the nervous system.

■ USE

When buying walnuts, choose nuts in their shells.
They keep better and have not begun the rotting process like those that are already shelled.
The walnut is actually quite fragile when in contact with air.

■ PRECAUTIONS

Eaten in excess, the walnut is difficult to digest.
It can also cause sores in the mouth and some allergies.

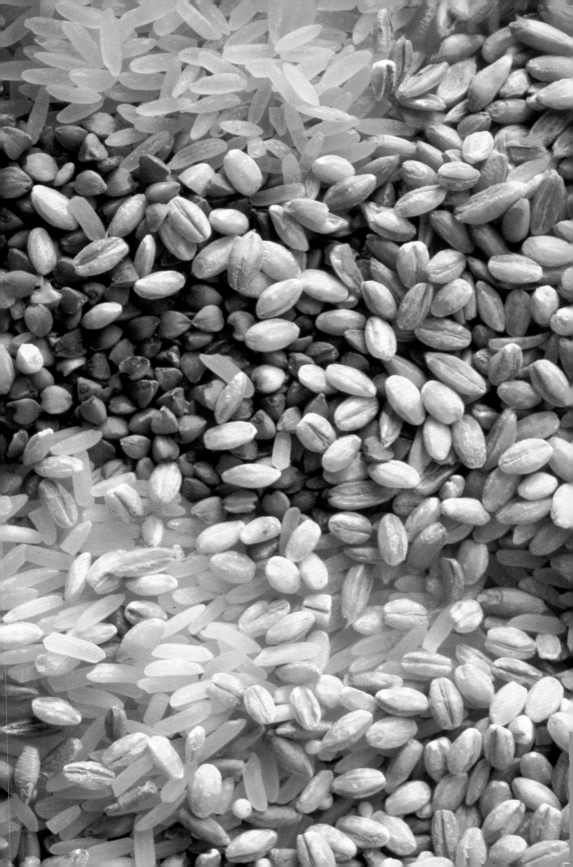

WHEAT

LOWERS BAD CHOLESTEROL.

■ ACTIVE INGREDIENTS

Wheat (especially if it is whole wheat) contains vitamins B and E, minerals and trace elements, such as phosphorus, magnesium, iron, zinc, manganese, selenium.

Whole wheat contains about 15% bran. This is the envelope that disappears during the refining process.

■ PROPERTIES

Wheat (especially wheat germ) promotes the reduction of «bad»cholesterol.

Whole wheat promotes intestinal transit, and would be part of foods that help fight cancer.

Whole wheat helps fight free radicals and cellular ageing.

■ PRECAUTIONS

Because of the presence of bran, wheat, in its complete form may irritate sensitive intestines.

Wheat is not suitable for people who are allergic to gluten, a protein present in this cereal.

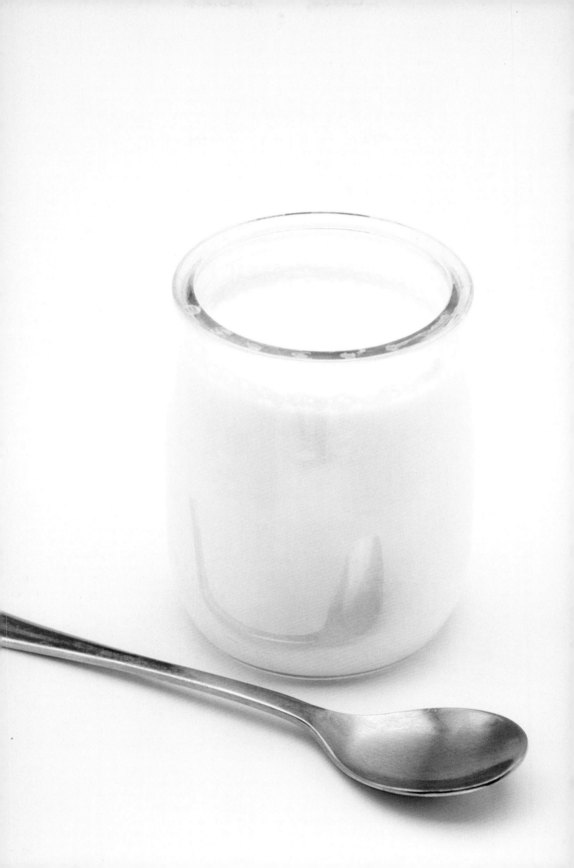

YOGHURT

FOR THE BALANCE OF THE INTESTINAL FLORA.

■ ACTIVE INGREDIENTS

Yogurt is a good source of protein. It contains lactic acid, lactobacilli bacteria, which allow the milk to ferment. Yogurt is rich in minerals, trace elements such as calcium, phosphorus, copper, zinc, and vitamin B.

■ PROPERTIES

Yogurt is more easily digested than milk.
It helps maintain and balance the intestinal flora.
It is helpful to the immune system.

■ USE

Yogurt will keep in the refrigerator. The "good to" date gives an indication as to when micro-organisms bear a sharp decline in vitality.
Thereafter, the yogurt is still edible for a very short time, but it has lost its properties. In general, yoghurt from sheep or goat milks is better tolerated and digested than cow's milk yoghurt.

■ PRECAUTIONS

People who are lactose intolerant should not consume yoghurt.

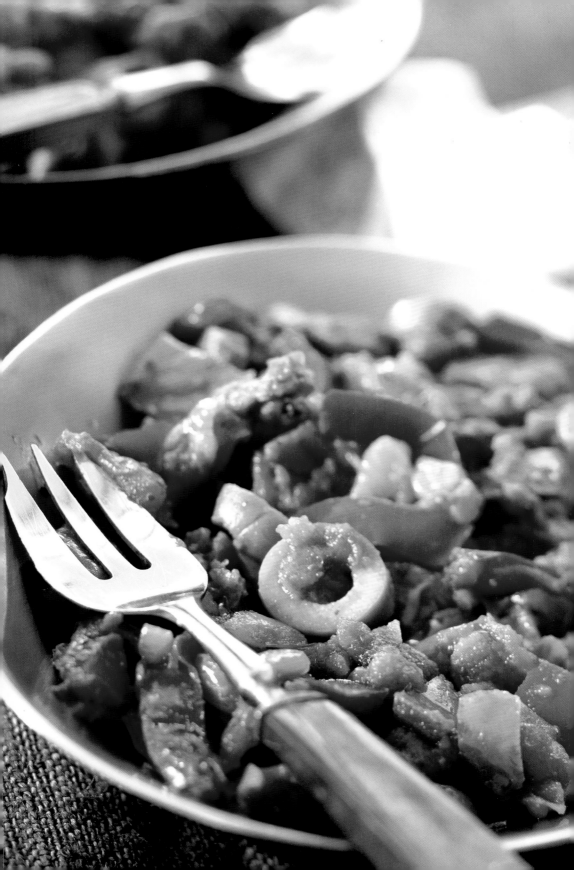

SOME RECIPES

GREEN "PUY" LENTILS

Easy. Preparation time: 10 minutes; cooking time: 35 minutes.

Ingredients for 4 persons:

- 300 g "Puy" lentils;

- spices: pepper (white, black and allspice)

- 3 tablespoons of olive oil.

- a few fresh leaves of white nettle (dead nettle);

- a few fresh leaves of mint.

1. Wash lentils and cook in salty water or in a light broth, skim and cover. Do not over-wet .

2. During cooking, prepare the olive oil (cold pressed), a mixture of pepper in a mill, turmeric, saffron, a little ground cumin, leaves fresh white nettle (dead nettle) and mint (if you don't have any, use an infusion of nettle and mint). Add all these ingredients, whose leaves have been chopped if they are fresh, to the lentils when lentils are cooked but slightly firm, make sure to leave little liquid so as not to get too dense a mass, but rather a slightly creamy mixture.

3. Adjust seasoning without being worrying too much about the oil content which, well chosen, will wonderfully flavor this dish.

(Recipe from Jean Cabodi, restaurateur, Dragon Inn, Limbour Belgium.)

SOME RECIPES

■ STEWED SWEET AND SOUR CARROTS WITH A SCENT OF CUMIN

Fairly difficult. Preparation time: 15 minutes; cooking time: 20 minutes.

Ingredients for 4 persons:

- 6 large carrots;
- 125 g of honey;
- 125 g of (apple) cider vinegar;
- 1 onion;
- spices: cumin and turmeric.

1. Peel and remove the ends of carrots before dicing, cut the onion in the same way.
Leave a medium saucepan to heat on your stove, then add a teaspoon of cumin, sauté one minute. Add honey, cider vinegar and the "tip of a knife-ful" of turmeric, and then add onions and carrots.

2. Leave to simmer until the carrot mixture and onions are slightly translucent. Remove from heat and eat warm or cold.

REUNION ISLAND GREAT CURRY

Very easy. Preparation time: 2hrs and 50mins.

Ingredients for 4 persons:

- 1 kg of pork loin;
- 2 red onions chopped;
- 2 cloves garlic, minced;
- 3 cm ginger, chopped;
- 1 bunch chopped cilantro;
- 1 shelf stock, poultry;
- 2 teaspoons curry powder;
- 4 tablespoon olive oil;
- salt and pepper;
- 4 tomatoes;
- 1 mango, not too ripe;
- 1 small spring onion;
- Juice of ½ a lime;
- 1 cucumber, peeled;
- a half bunch of mint, chopped;
- 2 velvety yogurt, small pots ;
- 1 tsp vinegar;
- 4 tablespoons vegetable oil;
- 1 tsp mustard;
- a pinch of pepper.

1. Cut the pork into small pieces. In a large skillet, place to heat the olive oil and brown the pork pieces over high heat.
Reduce to medium heat, remove the meat and add onions to cook, add ginger and garlic stirring often for 3-4 minutes.

2. Add the spices and turn again to cook one to two minutes.
Add meat and coat it with spices with a spoon.
Cover after adding water, season and add the stock cube.
Cook 2 hours at low heat. Meat should be tender.

3. While cooking, prepare the garnishes. Boil tomatoes, then peel them along with the onion.
Mix them with the ginger, spring onion and the juice of half a lemon. Salt, pepper and blend to a purée. Keep cool.

4. Remove seeds from cucumber and grate it. Mix it with yogurt and mint. Add salt and pepper and set aside to cool.

5. Make vinaigrette with the vinegar, mustard, salt, pepper, chili and oil.
Peel and chop mango into chunks, then toss with the vinaigrette.

6. Just before serving, add the coriander over the meat and serve with all the trimmings.

(Recipe Cyril Lignac, from the book "Petits Plats Exotiques".)

SOME RECIPES

◼ GARLIC SOUP

**Very easy. Preparation 20 minutes.
Cooking time 35 minutes.**

Ingredients for 6 persons:

- 700 g of potatoes;
- 3 heads of pink garlic ;
- 1 onion;
- 1 sprig of thyme;

- 20 cl of light cream;
- 5 cl of olive oil;
- 1 stock cube, salt, and pepper.

1. Peel and wash the potatoes, then cut them into cubes. Peel the garlic and chop onion.

2. Heat the oil in a saucepan and let onion and garlic melt for 5 minutes without letting their color change.

3. Pour 1.5 liters of cold water. Add diced potatoes, thyme, salt, pepper and stock cube.
Cover three quarters of pan with water and cook on medium heat for 30 minutes.

4. Mix the soup and add cream. Reheat gently before serving with croutons and sprinkle thyme.

■ LENTILS WITH SPINACH

Very easy. Preparation 10 minutes. Cooking time 35 minutes.

Ingredients for 4 persons:

- 200 grams of lentils;
- 400 g spinach;
- 1 large onion;
- 1 clove garlic;
- 2 tsp turmeric;
- 1 tsp ground cumin;
- 1 tsp ground cinnamon;
- 1 liter of water;
- 1 tablespoon olive oil;
- 1 lemon halved;
- salt and pepper.

1. Mince onion and garlic. Cook over low heat with spices in a pan with a little olive oil.

2. Add the lentils, water and salt. Bring to a boil, then reduce heat to low and simmer for 30 minutes, stirring.

3. In a pan, put to cook the spinach in a little water and salt. When ready, drain and set aside.

4. When lentils are cooked, mix them gently and add the spinach and mix them more roughly.

5. Add the juice of half a lemon and adjust seasoning.

SOME RECIPES

■ BASQUE "PIPERADE"

**Very easy. Preparation 10 minutes.
Cooking time 50 minutes.**

Ingredients for 6 persons:

- 6 small green chilies;
- 2 large onions;
- 4 cloves garlic;
- 3 green peppers;

- 6 tomatoes;
- 12 eggs;
- 150g Bayonne ham.

1. Remove seeds and peel the little green peppers and let parboil a few minutes in boiling water.

2. In a saucepan, pour a little oil and cook onions gently. Add the cloves of garlic mashed, green peppers and tomatoes cubed. Season and cook for 30 to 40 minutes until the tomatoes have given off their water.

3. Break the eggs into a bowl and beat them with a whisk.

4. Pour over the piperade and cook just long enough to get the eggs scrambled.

5. Golden the Bayonne ham on the pan and place it on the piperade.

6. Serve immediately with a little Espelette on top.

■ VEAL WITH PAPRIKA

Easy. Preparation 30 minutes, cooking 3 hours.

Ingredients for 4 persons:

- 800 g lean veal;
- 1 tablespoon mustard;
- 2 tsp paprika;
- ½ tsp marjoram;
- 100 g onions;

- 1 tspchopped parsley;
- 1 tbsp tarragon vinegar;
- 800 g carrots;
- 2 glasses of water, salt and pepper.

1. Peel and cut onion into small pieces. Then peel carrots and cut them into slices.

2. In a pot, pour the mustard that you dilute with water and the tarragon vinegar.

3. Add the herbs and spices, along with the pieces of veal which have been previously cut. Simmer over low heat for 3 hours.

SOME RECIPES

■ SAFFRON RISOTTO

Easy. Preparation 15 minutes - Cooking time 25 minutes.

Ingredients for 4 persons:

- 250 g risotto rice;
- 1 onion;
- ½ cup dry white wine;
- 1 bay leaf;
- 2 doses of saffron powder;
- 40 g margarine;
- salt and pepper.

1. Peel and finely chop the onion. Melt margarine over low heat. Add the onion and rice.
Sauté for 5 minutes without browning, stirring with a wooden spatula.

2. Pour the white wine and let evaporate over medium heat. Add salt, pepper, saffron powder and bay leaf. Pour 40 ml of hot water.
Cover and simmer 18 minutes over very low heat without stirring.

◼ ZAALOUK

Moderately easy. Preparation 15 minutes, cooking about 1 hour 10.

Ingredients for 4 persons:

- 1 kg of fresh tomatoes;
- 1 kg of medium eggplants;
- 15cl of olive oil;
- 3 cloves garlic;

- 4 tbsp chopped parsley
- 4 tbsp chopped cilantro
- 1 tsp ground cumin;
- salt, pepper

1. Preheat oven to 200 ° C (thermostat 6-7).
Brush tomatoes with a veil of olive oil. On two plates covered with aluminum foil, arrange the eggplants and tomatoes.
Bake for 30 minutes, the eggplant should be tender.

2. Remove vegetables from oven and let cool. Cut eggplants in half lengthwise. Remove the flesh with a spoon then chop. Remove skin and seed tomatoes, then mash the meat coarsely with a fork. Peel and crush the cloves of garlic with the flat part of a knife.

3. Sauté the tomato pulp and crushed garlic for 10 minutes
Add the eggplant flesh, parsley and chopped coriander/cilantro and salt and pepper.
Simmer uncovered for 20 minutes, stirring occasionally.
Add cumin after cooking and stir. Let cool, then keep in refrigerator.
Enjoy fresh.

SOME RECIPES

■ **CITRUS SALAD WITH SPICES**
Easy. Preparation time: 25 minutes.

Ingredients for 4 persons:

- 2 pomelos;
- 3 oranges;
- 1 lime;
- 2 tablespoons olive oil;

- a pinch of turmeric;
- a pinch of Espelette;
- a small piece of fresh ginge (about 2 cm).

1. Peel ginger and grate it finely.

2. Peel the pomelos and oranges using a sharp knife and removing completely the white part located under the skin

3. Slice oranges and pomelos and make a flower with the slices

4. Sprinkle with lime juice, pepper, turmeric and ginger.
Sprinkle a few drops of Olive oil. Serve at once to get the most from the vitamins.

WHITE CHOCOLATE STRAWBERRIES AND WASABI

Moderate difficulty. Preparation 30 minutes – cooking time 10 minutes; rest time: 1 hour.

Ingredients for 8 glasses:

- 300 g white chocolate
- 50 cl of cream,
- two sheets of gelatin;

Ganache:

- 140 g white chocolate
- 15 cl of cream,
- 15g of wasabi powder;

Strawberry puree:

- 400 g strawberries,
- 40 g sugar,
- juice of half a lemon.

1. For the mousse.
Soften gelatin in cold water. Bring 20 cl of liquid cream to a boil and let it dissolve the gelatin, then pour the mixture over white chocolate broken into small pieces.
Mix well and let stand for 10 minutes.
Whip the remaining liquid cream, then gently fold in whipped cream into white chocolate.
Fill the glasses to a third of their volume, and then put them in the refrigerator for at least 40 minutes.

2. For the ganache.
Mix the cream and wasabi in a saucepan and bring to a boil. Pour the mixture over white chocolate broken into small pieces and mix well. Garnish glasses with a thin layer of ganache and refrigerate for at least 20 minutes.

3. For the strawberry puree.
Rinse strawberries. Cut into small pieces and mash them lightly with a fork with icing sugar, lemon juice and 2 tablespoons of water to make a marmalade that's a little liquid. Just before serving, top with generous amounts of strawberry puree.

SOME RECIPES

■ **SPICED APPLES**

Moderate difficulty. Preparation time: 20 minutes Cooking time : 35 minutes.

Ingredients for 4 persons:

- 4 apples;
- 2 oranges;
- a pinch of cinnamon;
- half a vanilla bean;
- a star anise;

- a pinch of black pepper;
- 1 tbsp honey;
- 1 lemon;
- 4 sheets of parchment paper

1. Juice the oranges. Pour the juice into a small saucepan and add cinnamon, vanilla, star anise, pepper and honey.
Bring to a boil and reduce to half to get thick syrup. Remove the vanilla pod and star anise.

2. Preheat oven to 150 ° C (Gas 5).
Peel apples, core them and cut them in half. Wet them with lemon juice. Place two apple halves on a sheet of parchment paper, hollow side up.

3. Cover the apples with the orange syrup, and then close the "papilotte" of parchment paper. Do the same for all the apples.

4. Put in the oven for 20 minutes

Let stand in the oven for 5 minutes and enjoy warm.

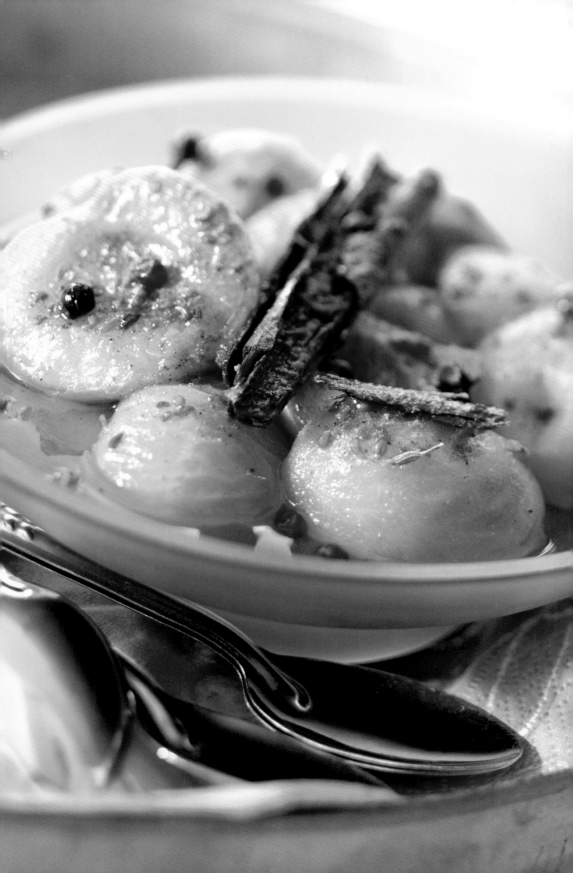

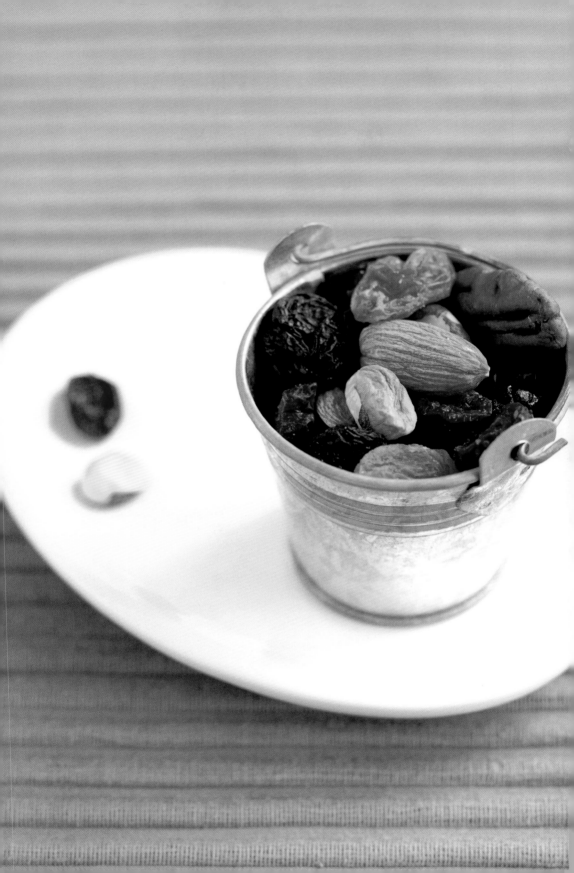

FOODS AND ILLNESSES

Allergy: cinnamon, lemon grass, cloves, tarragon, onion, nettle, horseradish, savory, tea.

Anemia: seaweed, lemon, watercress, strawberries, sprouts, kiwi, lentils, parsley, fish, pepper, orange, quinoa, grape, salad green tomato (flesh).

Anti-aging: seaweed, almonds, asparagus, avocado, broccoli, carrot, cherry, cilantro, watercress, turmeric, cabbage, raspberry, strawberry, seafood, nuts, beans, sprouts, kiwi fruit, oils Plant cold-pressed, lentils, miso, turnips, hazel, nuts, eggs, fish, pepper, apple, apple earth, plums, quinoa, raisins, soybeans, green tea, tomatoes, vinegar cider.

Arthritis: seaweed, asparagus, artichoke, celery, carrot, cabbage, lemon, turmeric, strawberries, wheat germ, currants, pumpkin seed oil, melon, turnip, apple, pear, grapes, tea, artichoke, apple cider vinegar.

Bloating (flatulence): dill, anise, basil, cardamom, caraway, celery, fennel, ginger, cold-pressed vegetable oils, lemon balm, mint, miso, fish, white rice, verbena, yogurt.

Cancer : garlic, seaweed, pineapple, asparagus, broccoli, carrot, black currant, whole grains, cabbage, lemon, watercress, strawberry seeds, sprouts, vegetable oils cold-pressed, miso, turnip, egg, onion, parsley, potato, pumpkin, quinoa, rhubarb, rye, soybeans, grapes, rice, green tea, tomato.

Cardiovascular disease: garlic, almonds, asparagus, broccoli, Cinnamon, whole grains, cabbage, lemon, chives, lemongrass, turmeric, spelled, seasonal fresh fruit, strawberry, dried fruit, ginger, cold pressed vegetable oil, fresh seasonal vegetables, legumes, lentils, mint, mustard, blueberry, hazelnut, walnut, onion, bitter orange, egg, pine nuts, pistachios, fatty fish, grape, licorice, rice, savory, rye, sesame, soybean, tea, tomato.

Cellulite: asparagus, basil, currants, celery, whole grains, cabbage, lemon, green vegetables, melon, blueberry, onion, watermelon, dandelion, pear, leek, apple, grape, green tea.

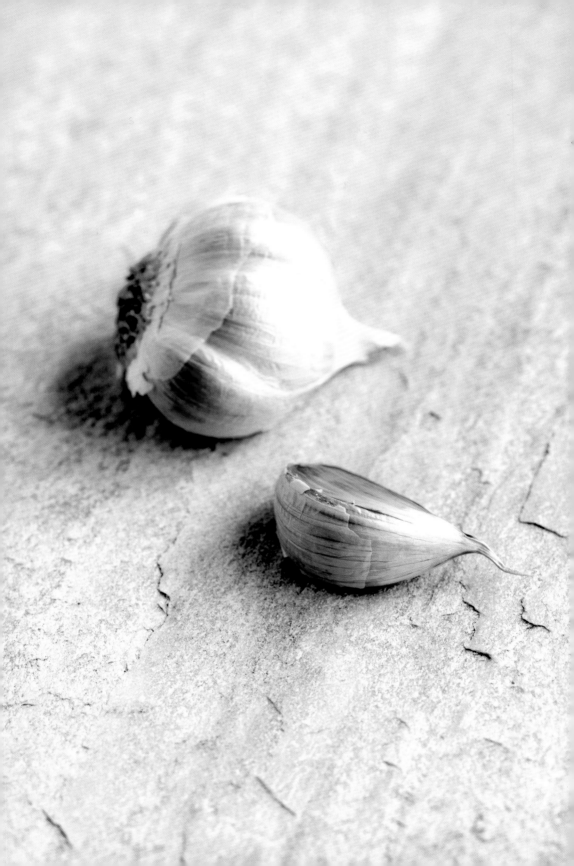

Cholesterol : garlic, seaweed, almonds, oats, chives, cloves, turmeric, tarragon, fresh seasonal fruit, seeds sprouts, cold-pressed vegetable oils, fresh seasonal vegetables, lentils, miso, walnut, nuts, onion, paprika, chickpeas, fish, potato, potato, pumpkin, radish, rice, soybean, tea, tomato, lean meat.

Colds: oats, carrot, lemon, fruit pulses, sprouts, ginger, honey, turnip, orange, barley, dandelion pepper, quinoa.

Constipation: seaweed, almond, artichoke, asparagus, eggplant, oats, whole wheat, whole grains, cabbage, squash, water, spelt, fennel, fig, strawberry, cold-pressed vegetable oils, kiwi, lentil, flax, corn, miso, turnips, walnuts, onion, orange, pearl barley, leek, potato, potato earth, plum, prune, grape, rice, rhubarb, salad, soy bran, tomato, artichoke.

Convalescence: seaweed, apricot, almond, oats, cinnamon, whole grain, chestnut, lemon, watercress, dates, spelt, fig, ginger, sprouts, cold-pressed vegetable oils, honey, millet, miso, nut, nuts, orange, fish, potato, potato, quinoa, wild rice

Cough: Garlic, anise, basil, chestnuts, cabbage, quinces, eucalyptus, fennel, ginger, lettuce, honey, mustard, turnip, onion, sorrel, parsley, radishes, grapes, thyme.

Cystitis: garlic, cranberries, asparagus, capers, celery, chervil, cherry, cabbage, lemon, water, currants, mint, honey, blackberry, blueberry, turnip, onion, nettle, dandelion, pear, leek, horseradish, sesame.

Diarrhea: garlic, artichoke, banana, cinnamon, carrot, chestnut, lemon, quince, miso, blueberry, onion, apple, potato, white rice vinegar, cider, yogurt.

Fatigue: apricot, seaweed, almonds, artichokes, oats, banana, basil, coffee, cinnamon, carrot, cloves, chestnuts, cabbage, whole grains, citrus, watercress, figs, ginger, cloves, sprouted seeds, vegetable oils Trial cold-pressed, lentils, mint, honey, millet, egg, orange, barley, fish, potato, potato, quinoa, raisins, salads, savory, rosemary, sage, sesame, tea, thyme, vanilla, meat, cider vinegar, yogurt.

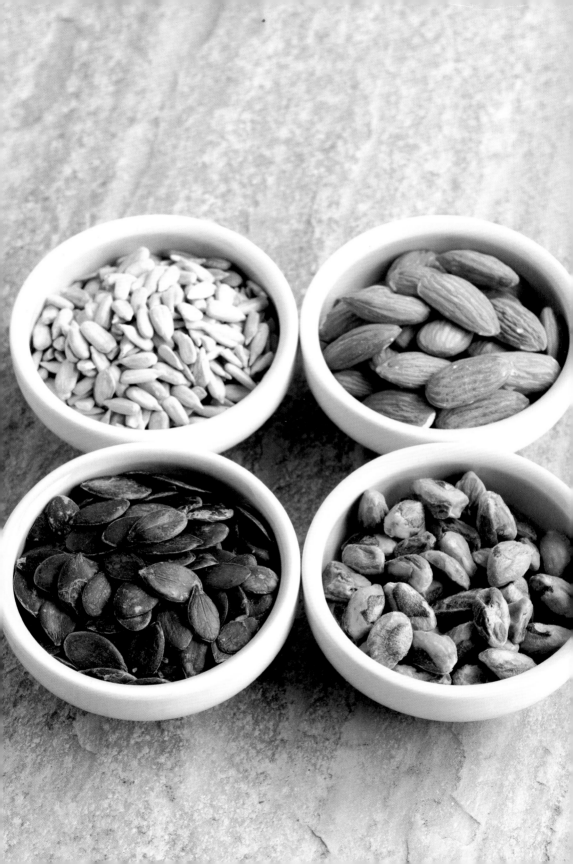

Fever: garlic, cinnamon, lemon, eucalyptus, mint, honey, blueberry, onion, barley, apples, sage, thyme, verbena.

Hepatic problems: artichoke, avocado, cabbage, strawberry, currant, vegetable oils cold-pressed, honey, nuts, papaya, parsley, dandelion, potatoes, radishes, grapes, rosemary, sage, Jerusalem artichoke.

Immune system: garlic, cranberry, pineapple, artichoke, avocado, carrot, cabbage, lemon, watercress, spelled, figs, dried fruit, ginger, clove, sprouts, cold-pressed vegetable oils, kiwi, linseed, mango, honey, blueberry, onion, hazelnuts, walnuts, grapefruit, apple, oily fish, peppers, quinoa, rice, sesame, soy, green tea, tomato, yogurt.

Indigestion: agar-agar, dill, anise, basil, cinnamon, capers, cardamom, caraway, chervil, chives, lemon, lemongrass, cloves, coriander, cumin, turmeric, spelt, tarragon, sprouts, ginger, bay leaves, mint, millet, miso, nutmeg, onion, paprika, pepper, licorice, apple, potato, saffron, savory, sage, sesame, rice, artichoke.

Inflammation (swelling): asparagus, oats, carrots, black currant, cherry, cabbage, cranberries, turmeric, fennel, bilberry, barley, apples, rhubarb, sage, thyme.

Influenza: garlic, oats, lemon, fennel, onion, grapefruit, sage, thyme, cider vinegar.

Intestinal gas: garlic, pineapple, celery, cinnamon, cardamom, tarragon, fennel, mint, miso.

Menopause: almond, pineapple, seaweed, oats, broccoli, celery, whole grains, cabbage, watercress, cumin, cheese, seeds sprouts, beans, cold pressed vegetable oil, kiwi, green vegetables, lentils, hazelnuts, walnuts, onion, potato, quinoa, sage, sesame, soybean, rice, yogurt.

Migraine: basil, lemon, ginger, mint, soy.

Motion sickness: lemon, ginger, mint, parsley, cider vinegar.

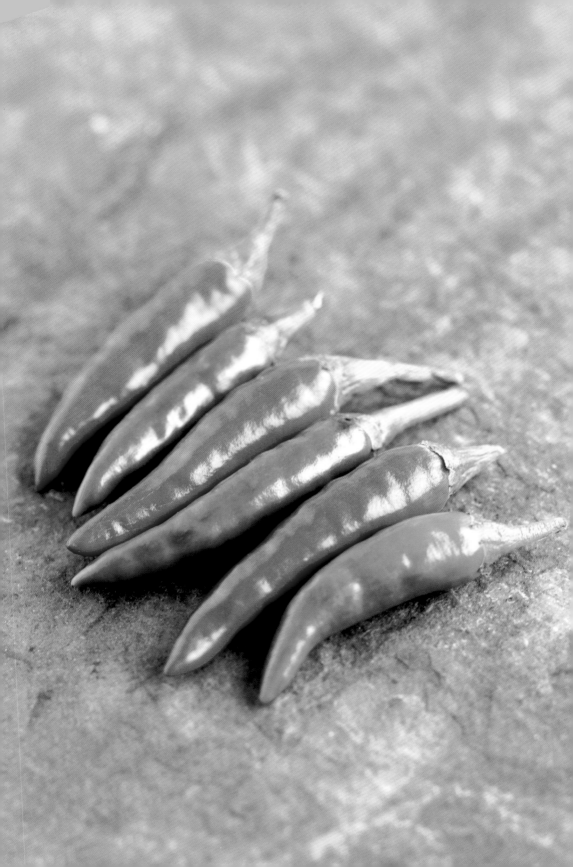

Nails: garlic, almonds, whole grains, cabbage, cheese, nuts, vegetable oils cold-pressed, kiwi, lentil, egg, fatty fish, potatoes, grapes, soybeans, yogurt.

Osteoarthritis: artichoke, broccoli, cherries, cauliflower, cabbage, kohlrabi, dates, strawberry, raspberry, cold pressed vegetable oils flaxseed, blueberry, turnips, nuts, fish, pepper, radish, soybean, cider vinegar.

Osteoporosis: garlic, seaweed, broccoli, cabbage, watercress, spinach, fig, raspberry, cheese, dried fruit, sprouts, lentils, egg, barley, quinoa, parsley, buckwheat, sesame, soy yogurt. `

Prostate: Avocado, whole grains, cabbage, pumpkin, seeds sprouts, beans, cold pressed vegetable oil, lentil, flax, onions, pumpkin seeds, parsley, fish fat, soybean, tomato.

Rheumatism: garlic, anise, carrot, capers, currants, celery, cherries, cabbage, lemon, turmeric, cloves, strawberry, ginger, currants, cold pressed vegetable oil , kiwi, mint, honey, nutmeg, egg, onion, nettle, dandelion, oily fish, apple, rosemary, sage, thyme, cider vinegar.

Sleep (difficulty): almond, avocado, banana, basil, broccoli, whole grains, cabbage, cilantro, watercress, tarragon, sprouts, vegetable oils Trial cold-pressed, lettuce, lemon balm, honey, hazelnut, walnut, onion, fish, potato, rosemary, saffron, soy, lime, artichoke, verbena yogurt.
`

Slimming down: seaweed, asparagus, whole grains, citrus, fruits and vegetables in season, ginger, turnips, onion, paprika, pepper, dandelion, leeks, apples, tea, tomato, vanilla, cider vinegar.

Stress: citrus, almond, oats, bananas, watercress, Spelt, strawberry, fresh fruit, dried fruit, sprouts, millet, vegetable oils cold-pressed, kiwi, honey, miso, nuts, egg, fish, potato, quinoa, raisins, sesame seeds, yogurt

Vision: apricot, garlic, cranberry, broccoli, carrot, black currant, cherry, cabbage, Lemon, spinach, blueberry, orange, grapefruit, pepper, tea

Water retention: seaweed, asparagus, artichoke, celery, chervil, cherry, lemon, cucumber, fennel, strawberry, gin, melon, blueberry, onion, barley, watermelon, dandelion, Pear, leek, apple, plum, grape, tea, apple cider vinegar.

GLOSSARY

Aldéhyde : lAldehyde: liquid made from alcohol by oxidation.

Antioxidant: substance that preserves tissue damage caused by reactive forms of oxygen, in which we count the free radicals.

Benign prostate hypertrophy: This development of the natural volume of the prostate can sometimes cause bothersome symptoms. In industrialized countries such as the USA, affects more than a million men over 50 years of age.

Benzodiazepines: root chemical being part of the composition of many tranquilizer products.

Bloat: accumulation of gas in the digestive tract, generating a distension of the stomach, leading to discomfort and sometimes pain (bloating).

Camphor: aromatic substance with antiseptic and anesthetic properties A cardiac and respiratory stimulant.

Carminative: favoring the expulsion of intestinal gas.

Essential oil: a substance extracted from volatile liquids secreted by herbs.

Eugenol: substance present in certain plants, with analgesic and disinfectant properties.

Flavonoids: a class of compounds synthesized by plants fruits, and vegetables in general.

Neolithic: a prehistoric era marked by deep technological and social change linked to the adoption by human groups of a production economy based on agriculture and livestock, and most often involving settlement.

Oxidative stress: responsible for the ageing of all organic tissue and a pivotal mechanism responsible for degenerative pathologies whose incidence increases with age.

Phytoestrogens: a substance synthesized by plants whose structure is close to female hormones.

Terpene: generic name for plant hydrocarbons (plant oils)

Also available at Alpen éditions

The Diet & Cookbooks Series:
Montignac Diet Cookbook
Montignac French Diet for Weight Loss
Eat Yourself Slim
Food Healing
Forever Young
The Anti Cholesterol Diet
The French GI Diet for Women
Osteoarthritis, Rheumatism, Arthritis

The Health books Series:
All About the Prostate
Control your Acidity: The Acid-Base Diet
Handle your Menopause
Herbal Healing
Living with a Hyperactive Child
Montignac Glycemix Index Diet
Omega-3 Answer
Osteoporosis
The French Paradox
The Paleo Diet
The XXL Syndrome

www.alpen.mc

A healthy balanced diet is certainly a key to enablin
us to stay fit and enjoy good health all through life.

It would seem that Americans care more and about the quality of what's
their plate.

Indeed, if inadequate or excessive intake of some nutrients may be the cau
of certain diseases, intake of «good» foods may be the smartest strategy
the fight against many health problems.

And faced with the difficulties we may feel when we're trying to sort out th
wealth of information often contradictory that is given to us daily, let's n
throw in the towel.

Healthy foods are available to us and really, we do not need too much food
maintain a good capital (of) health; we just need to know what to eat.

For each food, you will find:

- **its nutritional characteristics/value**
- **properties**
- **possible precautions**

*Elizabeth Brette is a biochemist who has worked at the Nice hospital in France
for 15 years.*

*A naturopath, Alessandra Moro Buronzo lives in Paris where she has worked
for the past 18 years.*

www.alpen.mc

ISBN: 978-23593

9 782359 340

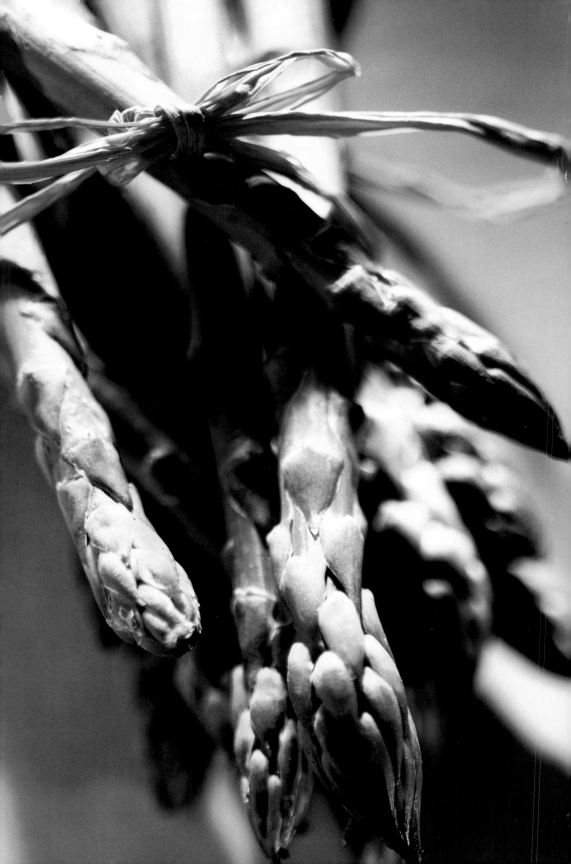